Prentice Hall Health's

Q&A Review

Massage Therapy

Third Edition

Jane S. Garofano, PhD, NCTMB

Owner/Director
JSG School of Massage Therapy

Associate Professor of Biological Sciences
Bergen Community College
Paramus, New Jersey

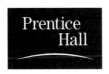

Prentice
Hall

Upper Saddle River, New Jersey

Library of Congress Cataloging-in-Publication Data
Garofano, Jane Schultz
Prentice Hall Health's question and answer review of massage therapy / Jane S. Garofano.— 3rd ed. p. cm.
Previously published under the title: Therapeutic massage & bodywork.
Includes bibliographical references.
ISBN 0-13-049098-9
1. Massage therapy—Examinations, questions, etc. I. Garofano, Jane Schultz.
Therapeutic massage and bodywork. II. Title.
RM721 .G34 2004
615.8'22'076—dc21

2002029822

Notice: The author[s] and the publisher of this volume have taken care that the information and technical recommendations contained herein are based on research and expert consultation, and are accurate and compatible with the standards generally accepted at the time of publication. Nevertheless, as new information becomes available, changes in clinical and technical practices become necessary. The reader is advised to carefully consult manufacturers' instructions and information material for all supplies and equipment before use, and to consult with a healthcare professional as necessary. This advice is especially important when using new supplies or equipment for clinical purposes. The author[s] and publisher disclaim all responsibility for any liability, loss, injury, or damage incurred as a consequence, directly or indirectly, of the use and application of any of the contents of this volume.

Publisher: Julie Levin Alexander
Assistant to Publisher: Regina Bruno
Senior Acquisitions Editor: Mark Cohen
Assistant Editor: Melissa Kerian
Editorial Assistant: Mary Ellen Ruitenberg
Senior Marketing Manager: Nicole Benson
Marketing Assistant: Janet Ryerson
Product Information Manager: Rachele Strober
Director of Manufacturing and Production: Bruce Johnson
Production Managing Editor: Patrick Walsh
Production Liaison: Alex Ivchenko
Production Editor: Amy Hackett, Carlisle Publishers Services
Manufacturing Manager: Ilene Sanford
Manufacturing Buyer: Pat Brown
Design Director: Cheryl Asherman
Senior Design Coordinator: Maria Guglielmo Walsh
Cover Design: Janice Bielawa
Manager of Media Production: Amy Peltier
New Media Project Manager: Stephen Hartner
Composition: Carlisle Publishers Services
Printing & Binding: Banta Harrisonburg
Cover Printer: Coral Graphics

Pearson Education LTD.
Pearson Education Australia PTY, Limited
Pearson Education Singapore, Pte. Ltd.
Pearson Education North Asia Ltd.
Pearson Education Canada, Ltd.
Pearson Educación de Mexico, S.A. de C.V.
Pearson Education — Japan
Pearson Education Malaysia, Ptc. Ltd.

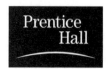

10 9 8 7 6 5
0-13-049098-9

*This book is dedicated to my family: Neil, Julie, Paul, and Mom,
who encouraged me to continue to write.*

A special thanks to all my pets for their company.

Contents

Preface

Prentice Hall Health's Question and Answer Review of Massage Therapy, 3rd Ed. has been designed and revised according to the guidelines of the National Certification for Therapeutic Massage and Bodywork (NCTMB) exam, which is administered throughout the United States, Canada, and Puerto Rico. This review book enables the applicant to review relevant material while becoming familiar with the types of questions given on the exam. Each question has one answer and a brief explanation with references provided at the end of each chapter. The questions are divided into four chapters that cover all areas of therapeutic massage and bodywork and closely correlate in percentage to the NCTMB exam content areas outlined in the *NCTMB Candidate Handbook.* The content is divided into Human Anatomy, Physiology, and Kinesiology (27%); Massage Therapy and Bodywork Theory, Assessment, and Practice (41%); Clinical Pathology and Recognition of Various Conditions (20%); and Professional Standards, Ethics, and Business Practices (12%) for a total of 600 questions. Within these content areas, additional topics relevant to non-Western bodywork and holistic touch-therapy modalities as well as ethics and clinical pathology are included and outlined below.

I. Human Anatomy, Physiology, and Kinesiology (27%)

  A. Western

    1. Major systems: location and function
   - Integumentary system
   - Skeletal system
   - Muscular system
   - Nervous system
   - Endocrine system
   - Cardiovascular system
   - Lymphatic and immune system
   - Respiratory system
   - Digestive system
   - Urinary system
   - Reproductive system
   - Craniosacral system

    2. Biomechanics and kinesiology
   - Efficient and safe movement patterns
   - Proprioception

- Basic principles of biomechanics and kinesiology
  3. Basic medical terminology
  B. Non-Western
  1. Traditional Chinese medicine
     - Primary meridians and organ physiology
     - Extraordinary meridians—conception and governing vessels
     - Five element theory
  2. Other energetic systems

II. Clinical Pathology and Recognition of Various Conditions (20%)
  A. History and client intake process
    1. Emotional states and stress leading to disease
    2. History of abuse and trauma related to disease and recovery
    3. Impact of client medical history on disease and recovery
    4. Effects of life stages on basic health and well-being
  B. Disease and injury-related conditions
    1. Signs and symptoms of disease of the major systems of the body: indications and contraindications
    2. Physiological changes and healing mechanisms

III. Massage Therapy and Bodywork Theory, Assessment, and Practice (41%)
  A. Assessment
    1. Effects of gravity
    2. Integration of structure and function
    3. Use of palpation for assessment of craniosacral pulses, energy blockages, and bony landmarks
    4. Somatic holding patterns in clients
    5. Using visual cues in assessing clients
    6. Conventional Western medical approaches to client's illness
    7. Structural compensatory patterns
    8. Interview techniques
  B. Application
    1. Sites to avoid on client's body
    2. Proper client draping and positional support

3. Physiological and emotional effects of touch on client
4. Effective and appropriate responses to client's emotional needs
5. Universal precautions
6. Use of appropriate verbal and nonverbal communication skills
7. Physiological changes brought about by touch therapy
8. Practitioner's self-awareness during a session
9. Using strategies to plan single and multiple client sessions
10. Use of manual contact and manipulation to affect soft tissue, joints, and the energy system
11. Use of joint mobilization techniques
12. Use of terms related to quality of movement
13. Using and teaching basic principles of posture and kinesthetic awareness
14. Hydrotherapy
15. CPR and first aid

IV. Professional Standards, Ethics, and Business Practices (12%)
  A. NCTMB Code of Ethics
  B. Confidentiality of client information
  C. Effective interprofessional communication
  D. Use of proper income-reporting procedures
  E. Basic business and accounting practices
  F. Session record-keeping practices
  G. Scope of practice: legal and ethical parameters

The last section of the review book contains a Comprehensive Simulated Exam of 150 questions selected from the previous bank of questions and answers. There are 150 multiple choice questions also available on the CD-ROM packaged with this book. The exam is given by an electronic testing system; therefore, the CD-ROM is included to practice the test on a computer in the three-hour period provided at the testing center. The answer key and rationales follow.

The reference list includes books recommended by the NCBTMB, as well as a few additional resources that include recent and relevant material that should be referred to during review.

Jane S. Garofano

Introduction

SUCCESS ACROSS THE BOARDS: THE PRENTICE HALL HEALTH REVIEW SERIES

Prentice Hall Health is pleased to present *Success Across the Boards,* our new review series. These authoritative texts give you expert help in preparing for certifying examinations. Each title in the series comes with its own technology package, including a CD-ROM and a Companion Website. You will find that this powerful combination of text and media provides you with expert help and guidance for achieving success across the boards. This question and answer review of massage therapy provides help for preparing for the National Certification for Therapeutic Massage and Bodywork exam (NCTMB).

COMPONENTS OF THE SERIES:

The series is made of a book and CD-ROM.

QUESTION AND ANSWER REVIEW OF MASSAGE THERAPY BY JANE S. GAROFANO

- **Content Review:** Key topics covered on the NCTMB exam are included in this book. This book has been designed to help the student review massage therapy and bodywork. Six hundred multiple choice questions are organized by the topics covered on the NCTMB exam and follow the exam format to a large extent. Working through these questions will help you assess your strengths and weaknesses in each topic of study. Correct answers and rationales are included. All questions are referenced to related textbooks so that you can quickly and easily find resources for more in-depth explanation or study on a specific topic.
- **Practice Exam:** A Comprehensive Simulated Practice test with 150 questions is included at the end of the book. This exam represents the content contained in the NCTMB exam, that is,

  1. Anatomy, Physiology, and Kinesiology
  2. Massage Therapy and Bodywork Theory, Assessment, and Practice
  3. Clinical Pathology and Recognition of Various Conditions
  4. Professional Standards, Ethics, and Business Practices

This test will give you a chance to experience the exam before you actually have to take it. Three hours are allowed for examination time.

- **About the CD-ROM:** A CD-ROM is included in the back of this book. The accompanying CD provides 300 additional practice multiple-choice questions and a glossary to help you learn definitions of key terms. Two tests each contain 150 questions based on the content code and their percentages as outlined in the *NCTMB Candidate Handbook.* Correct answers and comprehensive rationales and references follow all questions. You will receive immediate feedback to identify your strengths and weaknesses in each topic covered.

CERTIFICATION

The National Certification Board for Therapeutic Massage and Bodywork (NCBTMB) is a nationally recognized credentialing body formed to set standards for those who practice therapeutic massage and bodywork.

The NCBTMB developed and adopted the Standards of Practice to provide a clear statement of the expectations of professional conduct and level of practice afforded the public in, among other things, the following areas: Professionalism, Legal and Ethical Requirements, Confidentiality, Business Practices, Roles and Boundaries, and Prevention of Sexual Misconduct.

To contact the Board of Certification for a *NCTMB Candidate Handbook* please write, call, or send e-mail to:

National Certification Board for Therapeutic
    Massage and Bodywork
8201 Greensboro Drive
Suite 300
McLean, VA 22102
1-800-296-0664 or 703-610-9015
www.ncbtmb.com

QUALIFICATIONS FOR THE CERTIFIED MASSAGE THERAPIST

There are two ways that a student is eligible to take the certifying exam. Each method requires specific amounts of training and/or experience as a therapeutic massage and/or bodywork professional. The eligibility methods are the Education/Training Process and the Portfolio Review Process.

EDUCATION/TRAINING PROCESS

- Candidates must have graduated with at least 500 in-class hours of formal training at an accredited school of massage and/or bodywork.
- The formal training must be from a state-licensed training institute.
- Proof of graduation from a formal training program. This proof is in the form of an official school transcript and a notarized copy of the diploma or certificate of completion.

PORTFOLIO REVIEW PROCESS

The Portfolio Review Process lets the candidate put a portfolio together of all their training experience to be reviewed by an Eligibility Committee. This committee is made up of experienced massage therapy and bodywork practitioners and determines if the portfolio is equivalent to 500 hours of training.

ABOUT THE EXAM

The exam is given on an electronic testing system. The EXPro system does not use paper and pencil answer sheets. Instead, exam questions and options are displayed on a touch-sensitive screen. A computer memory card records the responses and automatically times the exam. EXPro lets the user change their answers, skip questions and marks questions for later review.

Before starting the exam, a tutorial may be taken to become familiar with how to use the EXPro system. This time is not taken away from the three hours allotted for the exam. The exam will be scored upon completion so the results will be immediately available.

The exam does not cover any specific method of massage and/or bodywork in depth. Instead, it covers the knowledge and skills that are common among all massage and/or bodywork disciplines. It also covers the basic approaches of Western and non-Western massage and/or bodywork.

The exam is divided into four basic areas: Human Anatomy, Physiology, and Kinesiology (27%); Massage Therapy and Bodywork Theory, Assessment, and Practice (41%); Clinical Pathology and Recognition of Various Conditions (20%); and Professional Standards, Ethics, and Business Practices (12%). The exam has 170 multiple-choice questions. Twenty of these questions will not be counted when the exam is scored. These questions are the pretest questions that are randomly distributed throughout the exam. The test taker does not know which items are the pretest questions and which are not. All questions should be answered.

Four distracters are provided for each question. Only one of the four answer choices is correct. There is no penalty for guessing. There are three hours allotted to complete the exam. The computer scores the exam as either "passing" or "failing."

STUDY TIPS

REVIEW MATERIALS

Choose review materials that contain the information you need to study. Save time by making sure that you aren't studying anything you don't need to. Before the exam, the best study preparation would be to use this question and answer review to identify your strengths and weaknesses. The references at the end of each rationale (i.e., in the Answers and Discussion Sections) will direct you to additional resources for more in-depth study.

Before attempting the questions in the review book, a thorough knowledge of anatomy and physiology is essential, particularly of the bones, muscles, blood vessels, and nerves. All methods of therapeutic massage and bodywork, including individual strokes and meridians, as well as prominent people that are associated with the methods, are important to know. It is also necessary to have an understanding of the ethical and business philosophies. Review draping techniques and personal hygiene. Be familiar with the ailments, injuries, and diseases that can benefit from therapeutic massage and how to treat them along with any first aid needed. A reference list is included as a guide to study specific areas.

We believe that you will find the questions, explanations, and format of the text to be of great as-

sistance to you during your review. We wish you luck on the exam.

SET A STUDY SCHEDULE

Use your time-management skills to set a schedule that will help you feel as prepared as you can be. Consider all the relevant factors: the materials you need to study, how many months, weeks, or days until the test date, and how much time you can study each day. If you establish your schedule ahead of time and write it in your date book, you will be much more likely to follow it.

TAKE PRACTICE TESTS

Practice as much as possible, using the questions in this book, and on the accompanying CD. These questions were designed to follow the format of questions that appear on the exam you will take, so the more you practice with these questions, the better prepared you will be on test day.

The printed practice test in the back of the book and the practice tests on the CD will give you a chance to experience the exam before you actually have to take it and will also let you know how you're doing and where you need to do better. For best results, we recommend you take a practice test 2 to 3 weeks before you are scheduled to take the actual exam. Spend the next weeks targeting those areas in which you performed poorly by reviewing questions in those areas.

Practice under test-like conditions, that is, in a quiet room, with no books or notes to help you, and with a clock telling you when to quit. Try to come as close as you can to duplicating the actual test situation.

TAKING THE EXAMINATION

PREPARE PHYSICALLY

When taking the exam, you need to work efficiently under time pressure. If your body is tired or under stress, you might not think as clearly or perform as well as you usually do. If you can, avoid staying up all night. Get some sleep so that you can wake up rested and alert.

Eating right is also important. The best advice is to eat a light, well-balanced meal before a test.

When time is short, grab a quick-energy snack such as a banana, orange juice, or a granola bar.

THE EXAM SITE

The exam site must be located prior to the required exam time. One suggestion is to find the site and parking facilities the day before the test. Parking fee information should be obtained so that sufficient money can be taken along on the examination day.

Allow plenty of time for travel to the site in case of unexpected mishaps such as traffic snarls. During travel, think positive thoughts (e.g., "My preparation for the exam was thorough, so I'll be able to answer the questions easily"). Maintain a confident attitude to prevent unnecessary stress.

MATERIALS

Be sure to take all required identification materials, registration forms, and any other items required by the testing organization or center. Read information and instructions supplied by the testing organizations thoroughly to be sure you have all necessary materials before the day of the exam.

READ TEST DIRECTIONS

Read the exam directions thoroughly! Because some board exams have different test sections with different question formats, it is important to be aware of changes in directions. Read each set of directions completely before starting a new section of questions.

SELECTING THE RIGHT ANSWER

Keep in mind that only one answer is correct. First read the stem of the question with *each* possible choice provided and eliminate choices that are obviously incorrect. Be cautious about choosing the first answer that *might* be correct; all possibilities should be considered before the final choice is made; the best answer should be selected.

If a question is complicated, try to break it down into small sections that are easy to understand. Pay special attention to qualifiers such as *only, except,* and so on. For example, negative words in a question can confuse your understanding of what the question asks ("Which of the following is *not. . .*").

INTELLIGENT GUESSING

If you don't know the answer, eliminate those answers that you know or suspect are wrong. Your goal is to narrow down your choices. Here are some questions to ask yourself:

- Is the choice accurate in its own terms? If there's an error in the choice, for example, a term that is incorrectly defined, the answer is wrong.
- Is the choice relevant? An answer may be accurate, but it may not relate to the essence of the question.
- Are there any distracters, such as *always, never, all, none,* or *every?* Qualifiers make it easy to find an exception that makes a choice incorrect.

Mark answers you aren't sure of, and go back to them at the end of the test.

Ask yourself whether you would make the same guesses again. Chances are that you will leave your answers alone, but you may notice something that will make you change your mind— a qualifier that affects meaning or a remembered fact that will enable you to answer the question without guessing.

WATCH THE CLOCK

Keep track of how much time is left and how you are progressing. Wear a watch or bring a small clock with you to the test room. A wall clock may be broken, or there may be no clock at all.

Some students are so concerned about time, that they rush through the exam and have time left over. In such situations, it's easy to leave early. The best approach, however, is to take your time. Stay until the end so that you can check your answers.

KEYS TO SUCCESS ACROSS THE BOARDS

- Study, review, and practice
- Keep a positive, confident attitude
- Follow all directions on the examination
- Do your best

Good luck!

You are encouraged to visit http://www.prenhall.com/success for additional tips on studying, test-taking and other keys to success. At this state of your education and career you will find these tips helpful.

Some of the study and test-taking tips were adapted from Keys to Effective Learning, Second Edition, by Carol Carter, Joyce Bishop, and Sarah Lyman Kravits.

Acknowledgments

I acknowledge the National Certification Board for Therapeutic Massage and Bodywork (NCBTMB) for setting high standards for massage and bodyworkers nationally and giving me the opportunity to write questions to improve skills as well as professionalism.

A sincere thank you goes to Prentice Hall's editorial staff, as well as Lois for the preparation and revision of the manuscript.

Reviewers

Gordie Blevins
Forsyth Tech Community College
Winston-Salem, North Carolina

Brett M. Carr, DC
Connecticut Center for Massage Therapy
Fairfield, Connecticut

Nancy W. Dail, BA, LMT, NCTMB
Downeast School of Massage
Waldoboro, Maine

Claire Doyle, MS, LMT
North Country Community College
Saranac Lake, New York

Randy Fillion, NCTMB, CTM
Irene's Myomassology Institute
Southfield, Michigan

Nancy Gamboian, PhD
Desert Institute of the Healing Arts
Tucson, Arizona

Dori L. Hess-Facemyer, MS, LMT, BS
Stark State College
Canton, Ohio

Meg Holloway, RN, MS, CMT
Johnson County Community College
Overland Park, Kansas

Janet Irene Wakefield, RN, CMT, NCTMB
Mountain State School of Massage
Charleston, West Virginia

Jerry Weinert, RN
Desert Institute of the Healing Arts
Tucson, Arizona

CHAPTER

1 Human Anatomy, Physiology, and Kinesiology

OBJECTIVES: Major areas of knowledge/content included in this chapter are based on the NCTMB exam topics and percentage of questions (27%)

1. Major systems: location and function

   - Integumentary
   - Skeletal
   - Muscular
   - Nervous
   - Cardiovascular
   - Lymphatic
   - Respiratory
   - Digestive
   - Urinary
   - Reproductive
   - Craniosacral

2. Biomechanics and kinesiology

   - Proprioception
   - Efficient and safe movement patterns

3. Medical terminology

4. Traditional Chinese medicine

   - Primary and extraordinary meridians
   - Five element theory

5. Other energetic systems

1. The tricuspid valve is found between the
   A. Right atrium and right ventricle
   B. Left ventricle and aorta
   C. Left ventricle and right ventricle
   D. Right atrium and left atrium

2. Which structure supports the body in the sitting position?
   A. Sacrum
   B. Coccyx
   C. Ischial tuberosity
   D. L5

3. Which statement is **TRUE** about the Golgi tendon apparatus?
   A. Found in joint capsules
   B. Detects overall tension in tendon
   C. Originates in Purkinje fibers
   D. Activated by vagel reflex

4. Which muscles are major adductors?
   A. Pectoralis and deltoid
   B. Pectoralis and latissimus dorsi
   C. Deltoid and latissimus dorsi
   D. Biceps and deltoids

5. Which supplies the lower limbs?
   A. Dorsal primary rami
   B. Sciatic nerve
   C. Lumbosacral plexus
   D. Femoral nerve

6. Which most accurately describes the meridian system?
   A. Energy pathway moving randomly through the body
   B. Energy pathway moving superficially
   C. Energy pathway that doesn't affect organs
   D. 12 meridians and 2 vessels are pathways in which energy moves toward the surface of the body, affecting organs

7. A holistic bodywork method that involves freeing the flow of energy through the body by using gentle rocking, the cradle, and an elbow milk is
   A. Acupressure
   B. Polarity therapy
   C. Reflexology
   D. Trager

8. The Conception Vessel is the confluence of all the
   A. Yin channels
   B. Yang channels
   C. Qi energy
   D. Five elements

9. The only joint in the upper body where the axial skeleton articulates with the appendicular skeleton is
   A. Sternoclavicular
   B. Glenohumeral
   C. Sternoscapular
   D. Scapularclavicular

10. Which muscle adducts and medially rotates the femur at the hip?
    A. Gluteus medius
    B. Pectineus
    C. Quadratus femoris
    D. Tensor fascia latae

11. Which muscle is closest to the sciatic nerve?
    A. Gracilis
    B. Piriformis
    C. Gluteus medius
    D. Pectineus

12. Which is the most important element to combat infection?
    A. RBCs
    B. Platelets
    C. WBCs
    D. Fibrinogen

13. Grounding exercises in shiatsu are important to prepare you by
    A. Connecting with the ground to remove tension
    B. Breathing correctly
    C. Increase awareness of your body weight
    D. All of the above

14. Acupuncture, shiatsu, polarity, and reflexology are examples of
    A. Energetic manipulation
    B. Behavioral barometer
    C. Reactive circuits
    D. Systematic massage

15. The movements at synovial joints include flexion/extension, abduction/adduction, and
    A. Rotation
    B. Isolation
    C. Dynamics
    D. Pivot

16. The finger pressure massage method called *shiatsu* is
    A. Japanese
    B. Chinese
    C. German
    D. French

17. When palming or massaging the medial side of the leg the following meridians are affected.
    A. BL, K, LI
    B. SP, Liv, K
    C. GB, Liv, Sp
    D. St, Sp, BL

18. Which of the following factors contribute to muscle fatigue?
    A. Insufficient oxygen
    B. Depletion of glycogen
    C. Lactic acid buildup
    D. All of the above

19. A sudden involuntary contraction of a muscle is called a (an)
    A. Levator
    B. Proximal
    C. Isometric
    D. Spasm

20. Which type of lever is characterized as having the fulcrum between the effort and resistance? An example is the head resting on the vertebral column.
    A. First class
    B. Second class
    C. Third class
    D. Fourth class

21. The energy flow of the Yin channels flow
    A. Finger tips to chest to feet
    B. Hand to head downward to the feet
    C. Head to hand downward to the feet
    D. Front of body and deep organs

22. Which facial muscle attaches into the mandible, angles of the mouth, and skin of the lower face?
    A. Buccinator
    B. Depressor labii inferior
    C. Levator labii superioris
    D. Platysma

23. What is the spinal nerve contribution that composes the brachial plexus?
    A. C_1–C_4; T_1
    B. C_5–C_8; T_1
    C. C_7–C_8; T_1
    D. T_2–T_{12}; L_1

24. The tools and techniques of Shiatsu include all but the following:
    A. Palming
    B. Thumbing
    C. Cross-fiber friction
    D. Stretches and rotation

25. Which of the following muscles are forearm flexors at the elbow joint?
  A. Biceps brachii, brachialis, triceps brachii
  B. Brachioradialis, anconeus, pronator quadratus
  C. Supinator, brachialis, biceps brachii
  D. Brachialis, brachioradialis, biceps brachii

26. Aligning major body segments through manipulation of connective tissue is the
  A. Rolfing method
  B. Trager method
  C. Palmer method
  D. Reflexology method

27. Which of the following does not flex the wrist?
  A. Flexor carpi radialis
  B. Flexor carpi ulnaris
  C. Pronator quadratus
  D. Palmaris longus

28. Which of the following is **NOT** a hamstring muscle?
  A. Adductor magnus
  B. Biceps femoris
  C. Semimembranosus
  D. Semitendinosus

29. What muscle forms the outer layer of the anterior and lateral abdominal wall?
  A. Rectus abdominis
  B. Transversalis
  C. Serratus anterior
  D. External oblique

30. The primary flexor of the distal phalanges of the fingers is
  A. Flexor carpi ulnaris
  B. Pollices longus
  C. Flexor digitorum profundus
  D. Flexor carpi radialis

31. During normal posture the body is in what type of contraction state?
  A. Tetanic
  B. Isotonic
  C. Isometric
  D. Tonic

32. Inguinal nodes serve the purpose of draining lymph from the
  A. Arm
  B. Lower neck
  C. Neck
  D. Leg

33. The energy for the stomach meridian is most effective from
  A. 7 AM to 9 AM
  B. 7 PM to 9 PM
  C. 3 AM to 5 AM
  D. 3 PM to 5 PM

34. The energy for the spleen meridian is most effective from
  A. 7 AM to 9 AM
  B. 7 PM to 9 PM
  C. 9 AM to 11 AM
  D. 11 PM to 1 AM

35. Muscle energy techniques (MET) include:
  A. Proprioceptive neuromuscular facilitation (PNF)
  B. Postisometric relaxation (PIR)
  C. Reciprocal inhibition (RI)
  D. All of the above

36. The membrane that surrounds the shaft of a long bone is the
  A. Synovial membrane
  B. Bursae
  C. Periosteum
  D. Peritoneum

37. With the elbow flexed, which muscle supinates the palm?

A. Pronator

B. Supinator

C. Quadrator

D. Brachialis

38. MET can be used to assess and stretch the piriformis muscle in the supine position by:

A. Rotating the knee laterally

B. Extending the knee to the chest

C. Adducting the knee over the opposite ASIS

D. Abducting the knee

39. The adductor muscles along the medial femoral region of the hip

A. Each has their origin on the pubic bone

B. Enhance hip flexion

C. Include the pectineus, adductor longus, brevis, magnus and gracilis

D. All of the above

40. Which of the following is **TRUE** about terminal ganglia?

A. They are also know as collateral ganglia

B. These ganglia receive sympathetic preganglionic fibers

C. These ganglia lie close to the vertebral column and the large abdominal arteries

D. These ganglia are located at the end of an autonomic motor pathway

41. In which directions do Yin meridians flow?

A. Superior to inferior

B. Inferior to superior

C. Lateral to medial

D. Medial to lateral

42. Which meridians are innervated when massaging the medial thigh?

A. KI, LIV, SP

B. GB, ST, SP

C. LIV, ST, KI

D. GB, LIV, KI

43. Which meridian has a point on the radial side of the little finger?

A. Small intestine

B. Triple warmer

C. Heart

D. Pericardium

44. The vascular system is controlled by which meridian?

A. Heart

B. Triple warmer

C. Pericardium

D. Conception vessel

45. Which meridian is involved with a system but does not have a corresponding organ?

A. Spleen

B. Heart

C. Liver

D. Triple heater

46. Which of the following moves an extremity away from the midline?

A. Adductor

B. Abductor

C. Flexor

D. Rotator

47. Which type of joints are found in the vertebrae?

A. Ball and socket

B. Gliding

C. Condyloid

D. None of the above

48. Which is a band of strong, fibrous tissue that connects the articular ends of bones and binds them together?

A. Tendon

B. Fascia

C. Cancellous tissue

D. Ligament

49. The blood type that is termed the "universal recipient" is
    A. O
    B. A
    C. B
    D. AB

50. An interosseous ligament of a syndesmosis area is located
    A. Near the articulation of a joint
    B. Between the radius and ulna to hold them together
    C. Around the patella bone
    D. Between the vertebrae

51. Which of the following points is located on the nail of the first toe?
    A. ST45
    B. KI1
    C. LIV1
    D. None of the above

52. The digestive organs drain into the
    A. Hepatic portal vein
    B. Aorta
    C. Vena cava
    D. Pulmonary artery

53. The elbow is proximal to the hand and the hand is _____ to the elbow.
    A. Medial
    B. Anterior
    C. Distal
    D. None of the above

54. Myelinated axon supported by neuroglia cells is
    A. White matter
    B. Gray matter
    C. Nucleus
    D. Ganglia

55. The _____ are the largest number of formed elements.

    A. Thrombocytes
    B. Leukocytes
    C. Erythrocytes
    D. Monocytes

56. Which meridians transverse the abdomen?
    A. BL, LU, TW
    B. HT, HC, LU
    C. GB, SI, CO
    D. KI, SP, ST

57. The plantar region is the most _____ of all the body regions.
    A. Distal
    B. Inferior
    C. Anterior
    D. Posterior

58. The radiocarpal joint is a (an)
    A. Hinge joint
    B. Ellipsoid joint
    C. Metacarpalphalangeal joint
    D. Pivot joint

59. Although the biceps brachii is the most visible flexor, another primary muscle is
    A. Brachialis
    B. Pronator quadratus
    C. Anconeus
    D. Triceps brachii

60. Where is the medial malleolus?
    A. Calcaneus
    B. Talus
    C. Fibula
    D. Tibia

61. The left coronary artery arises from the
    A. Ascending aorta
    B. Descending aorta
    C. Left atrium
    D. Left ventricle

62. Which part of a neuron carries impulses toward the cell body?
   A. Dendrite
   B. Axon
   C. Motor unit
   D. All of the above

63. The capitulum of the humerus articulates with the
   A. Radial tuberosity
   B. Head of the radius
   C. Olecranon of the ulna
   D. Coracoid

64. The median nerve is part of
   A. The sacral plexus
   B. Sciatic nerve
   C. Brachial plexus
   D. Lumbar plexus

65. Where are the first and last points on the BL meridian?
   A. Head and fingers
   B. Toes and fingers
   C. Head and foot
   D. Wrist and finger

66. Which muscle does the axillary nerve innervate?
   A. Deltoid
   B. Brachial
   C. Pectoralis major
   D. None of the above

67. The wrist and fingers can be extended by the
   A. Extensor carpi radialis, longus, brevis, extensor digitorum and ulnaris
   B. Brachioradialis
   C. Extensor carpi ulnaris and digitorum
   D. Extensor carpi radialis longus and brevis

68. Which is the **MOST** highly vascularized tissue?
   A. Muscle
   B. Ligament
   C. Nervous
   D. Tendon

69. Adult body temperature is higher than normal at
   A. 37° C
   B. 98° F
   C. 98.6° F
   D. 39° C

70. The triple warmer controls
   A. Assimilation, digestion, elimination
   B. Assimilation, digestion, skin temperature regulation
   C. Digestion, elimination, skin temperature regulation
   D. Elimination, digestion, nervous system

71. Which muscle abducts the scapula?
   A. Serratus anterior/pectoralis minor
   B. Rhomboids
   C. Latissimus dorsi
   D. Trapezius

72. Which is (are) not a part of the central nervous system (CNS)?
   A. Cranial nerves
   B. Cerebellum
   C. White tracts
   D. Medulla oblongata

73. The external iliac artery supplies blood to
   A. The lower limbs
   B. All parts of the trunk
   C. The neck and back
   D. The pelvic organs

74. What plantar flexes and everts the foot?
   A. Tibialis anterior
   B. Gastrocnemius
   C. Plantaris
   D. Peroneus longus

75. Manipulation of the sacral area **MOST** directly affects energy in which meridian?
    A. BL
    B. GNB
    C. KI
    D. ST

76. The normal resting pulse rate range is
    A. 70–80 beats per minute
    B. 80–90 beats per minute
    C. 120–130 beats per minute
    D. All of the above

77. Which muscle extends the femur?
    A. Soleus
    B. Gluteus minimus
    C. Gluteus maximus
    D. Peroneus

78. What is the normal systolic pressure?
    A. 80 mm/Hg
    B. 90 mm/Hg
    C. 120 mm/Hg
    D. 140 mm/Hg

79. The diaphragm contracts on
    A. Inspiration
    B. Expiration
    C. Both
    D. Neither

80. Lymph is interstitial fluid consisting of
    A. Water, cell debris, gases, metabolic wastes, bacteria
    B. Water and gas
    C. Blood, lymphocytes, bacteria
    D. Water alone

81. The nerve (s) that innervate the five flexor muscles of the forearm is (are)
    A. Radial
    B. Median
    C. Median and ulnar
    D. Radial and ulnar

82. A medial collateral ligament
    A. Connects the femur to the tibia
    B. Connects the femur to the fibula
    C. Crosses the middle of the knee joint
    D. Attaches to the anterior cruciate ligament

83. Which muscle is **NOT** part of the rotator cuff?
    A. Supraspinatus
    B. Infraspinatus
    C. Teres major
    D. Teres minor

84. The homeostatic responses of the body are regulated by which two systems?
    A. Digestive, urinary
    B. Reproductive, endocrine
    C. Endocrine, nervous
    D. Cardiovascular, respiratory

85. The most abundant inorganic substance in humans is
    A. Carbohydrate
    B. Lipid
    C. Oxygen
    D. Water

86. Which of the following is an acidic pH?
    A. 14
    B. 12
    C. 10
    D. 6

87. Good body mechanics is defined as
    A. Proper use of postural techniques
    B. Biomechanics to decrease fatigue
    C. Making use of the therapists body weight
    D. All of the above

88. The tendino-muscle channels of the lung pass through muscles of the chest and arm that include

A. Pectorals

B. Biceps brachii

C. Diaphragm

D. All of the above

89. In body mechanics the horse stance or warrior stance is used

    A. To perform short, traverse strokes, such as petrissage

    B. To perform long effleurage strokes

    C. To perform chair massage

    D. To adjust the massage table to the correct height

90. The governing vessel is the confluence of all the

    A. Yin channels

    B. Yang channels

    C. Qi energy

    D. Five elements

91. The epidermis is composed of

    A. Simple squamous epithelium

    B. Simple cuboidal epithelium

    C. Simple columnar epithelium

    D. Stratified squamous epithelium

92. Which of the following is **TRUE** about aging of the integumentary system starting with the late forties?

    A. Collagen fibers increase

    B. Elasticity increases in elastic fibers

    C. Fibroblasts decrease in number

    D. Hair and nail growth tends to speed up

93. A detailed map of the foot was developed by Ingham as *Zone Therapy* and later called

    A. Reflexology

    B. Polarity

    C. Amma therapy

    D. Shiatsu

94. What is the primary salt that makes bone matrix hard?

A. Calcium carbonate

B. Potassium chloride

C. Sodium chloride

D. None of the above

95. Which of the following processes forms a joint?

    A. Meatus

    B. Crest

    C. Tuberosity

    D. Condyle

96. Which of the following are paired cranial bones?

    A. Occipital and sphenoid

    B. Temporal and parietal

    C. Frontal and ethmoid

    D. Parietal and ethmoid

97. Which of the following is **TRUE** with regard to the humerus?

    A. The olecranon fossa is an anterior depression that receives the ulna's olecranon process

    B. The medial and lateral epicondyles are rough projections on either side of the proximal end

    C. The radial fossa is a posterior depression that receives the head of the radius when the forearm is flexed

    D. Its trochlea articulates with the ulna

98. The prominence felt on the medial surface of the ankle is the

    A. Fibular notch

    B. Medial condyle

    C. Medial malleolus

    D. Tarsus

99. The largest and strongest tarsal bone is the

    A. Calcaneus

    B. Cuboid

    C. Lateral cuneiform

    D. Navicular

100. Which of the following joint classifications is described as freely movable?
    A. Amphiarthrosis
    B. Cartilaginous
    C. Diarthrosis
    D. Fibrous

101. The joint between the trapezium carpal bone and the thumb's metacarpal is which kind of joint?
    A. Ball-and-socket
    B. Ellipsoidal
    C. Gliding
    D. Saddle

102. Which subtype of diarthrosis joint is found in the knee, elbow, and ankle?
    A. Ball-and-socket
    B. Ellipsoidal
    C. Gliding
    D. Hinge

103. Which of the following is an intra-articular ligament of the knee?
    A. Anterior cruciate
    B. Arcuate popliteal
    C. Medial collateral
    D. Oblique popliteal

104. Which of the following is **TRUE** concerning the microscopic anatomy of skeletal muscle?
    A. A sarcolemma is the muscle fiber's cytoplasm
    B. The skeletal muscle fiber is a long, cylindrical cell
    C. The sarcoplasma is the muscle fiber's plasma membrane
    D. Each skeletal muscle cell has several nuclei

105. The Ki flowing through the meridians is the
    A. Hara breathing meditation
    B. Blockage

C. Universal life energy
    D. Spirit

106. Jin Shin Do is an oriental therapy that is
    A. Preventative rather than symptomatic in nature
    B. To strengthen our absorption of life energy
    C. Acupressure, breathing and meditation
    D. All of the above

107. The Chinese consider the lung as the delicate organ because
    A. It is a delicate tissue
    B. It is the first organ to be injured by negative substances
    C. It cannot work without the heart
    D. All of the above

108. If a muscle is not used, the resulting condition is called
    A. Atrophy
    B. Myotrophy
    C. Hypertrophy
    D. Actintrophy

109. Which direction of muscle fiber is described as running parallel to the body's midline?
    A. Brevis
    B. Oblique
    C. Rectus abdominis
    D. Serratus

110. Which cheek muscle is a facial muscle?
    A. Buccinator
    B. Depressor labii inferioris
    C. Mentalis
    D. Platysma

111. At which vertebral level does the spinal cord end?
    A. First lumbar
    B. Between first and second lumbar

C. Fifth lumbar

D. Second sacral

112. Which of the following is **NOT** a functional component of a reflex arc?

A. Brain

B. Effector

C. Motor neuron

D. Receptor

113. Which reflex is essential to maintaining muscle tone and adjusts muscle performance during exercise?

A. Crossed extensor

B. Flexor

C. Stretch

D. Tendon

114. The deltoid muscle abducts the arm, and is often used as a site of injection. Which nerve stimulates it?

A. Axillary

B. Median

C. Musculocutaneous

D. Radial

115. The sciatic nerve is actually two nerves. Which nerves compose the sciatic nerve?

A. Common peroneal and pudendal

B. Tibial and medial plantar

C. Medial and lateral plantars

D. Common peroneal and tibial

116. Which of the following are involved in the abduction of the arm?

A. Deltoid and subscapularis

B. Supraspinatus and infraspinatus

C. Teres major and teres minor

D. Supraspinatus and deltoid

117. Which of the following are involved in the adduction of the arm?

A. Pectoralis major and latissimus dorsi

B. Infraspinatus and teres major

C. Teres minor and coracobrachialis

D. Pectoralis major, teres major, teres minor, latissimus dorsi, carica brachialis

118. Which of the following is **NOT** part of the erector spinae muscles?

A. Iliocostalis

B. Longissimus

C. Spinalis

D. Platysma

119. Which of the following muscles does **NOT** abduct the thigh?

A. Gluteus maximus

B. Gluteus medius

C. Gluteus minimus

D. Sartorius

120. Which of the following laterally rotates the thigh?

A. Obturator externus

B. Obturator internus

C. Piriformis

D. All of the above

121. Which of the following is the major muscle involved in crossing one's leg?

A. Gastrocnemius

B. Rectus femoris

C. Sartorius

D. Semimembranosus

122. The Amma therapy is a full-body manipulation of the coetaneous regions, twelve organ channels, governing and conception vessels as well as

A. Tendino-muscle channels

B. TS points

C. Yin-yang

D. Qi of the heaven

123. Which of the following statements about synaptic facts is **FALSE**?
   A. At a chemical synapse, only synaptic end bulbs of presynaptic neurons can release neurotransmitters
   B. Electrical synapses allow faster communication than do chemical synapses
   C. At a chemical synapse, ionic current spreads directly from one cell to another through gap junctions
   D. Presynaptic facilitation increases the amount of neurotransmitters released by a presynaptic neuron, whereas presynaptic inhibition decreases it

124. Which cranial nerve is incorrectly paired with its number?
   A. Olfactory–I
   B. Trigeminal–V
   C. Facial–VII
   D. Vestibulocochlear–X

125. Which of the following brain areas are thought to be associated with memory?
   A. Frontal lobe and temporal lobe association cortex
   B. Occipital lobe and parietal lobe association cortex
   C. Parts of the limbic system and diencephalon
   D. All of the above

126. The major role for initiating and controlling precise, discrete muscular movements comes from the
   A. Center of the thalamus
   B. Bulk of the hypothalamus
   C. Area lateral to the septum
   D. Motor portions of the cerebral cortex

127. An energy-balancing therapy that attempts to remove blockages and bring healing energy to the problem area is called
   A. Reflexology
   B. Therapeutic touch

C. Amma therapy
   D. Myofascial release

128. Which part of the brain regulates the balance of sympathetic versus parasympathetic activity?
   A. Hypothalamus
   B. Medulla
   C. Pineal gland
   D. Pons

129. When the dorsum of the foot is massaged, which meridians are stimulated?
   A. HT and KI
   B. LIV and SP
   C. LIV and KI
   D. All Yang meridians

130. Glucagon
   A. Accelerates the formation of glycogen from glucose (glycogenesis)
   B. Promotes glucose formation from lactate and certain amino acids
   C. Lowers the blood glucose level
   D. Does all of the above functions

131. Which of the following is **TRUE** about antidiuretic hormone (ADH)?
   A. During dehydration, ADH increases the rate of perspiration production
   B. Alcohol stimulates ADH secretion
   C. Pain, trauma, and anxiety suppress the secretion of ADH
   D. It is also called vasopressin

132. Blood pressure is lowest in
   A. Veins
   B. Capillaries
   C. Arteries
   D. Arterioles

133. Plasma constitutes what percentage of the blood?
   A. 20%

B. 40%

C. 55%

D. 45%

134. Blood carries

A. Carbon dioxide

B. Metabolic waste

C. Oxygen

D. All of the above

135. In the middle of the thoracic cavity is a space assigned to the heart called the

A. Pleural space

B. Pericardial space

C. Mediastinum

D. Sternal notch

136. A group of nerve cells that lie outside the CNS is called

A. Gray matter

B. White matter

C. Ganglia

D. Nucleus

137. The pulmonary circulation carries deoxygenated blood from the right ventricle to the air sacs of the lungs and returns oxygenated blood from the lungs to the

A. Right atrium

B. Left ventricle

C. Left atrium

D. Pulmonary valve

138. The first and largest branch of the arch of the aorta is the

A. Subclavian

B. Coronary

C. Carotid

D. Brachiocephalic

139. Within the brain, all veins drain into the

A. External jugular veins

B. Internal jugular veins

C. Vertebral veins

D. Cardiac veins

140. Lymph in the right leg would drain into the

A. Right lymphatic duct

B. Left thoracic duct

C. Cisterna chyli

D. B and C are correct

141. The Yin and Yang comprise a spiral of change that represents

A. Seasons

B. Life in constant flux

C. Rhythms in animals and man

D. All of the above

142. The end product of glycolysis is pyruvic acid, and its fate depends on

A. The body cellular need

B. The availability of oxygen

C. The transport in the bloodstream

D. All of the above

143. The mineral that is found in the hemoglobin of blood and that carries oxygen to body cells is

A. Phosphorous

B. Calcium

C. Magnesium

D. Iron

144. The Qi pathways or channels constitute the

A. Shiatsu vessels

B. Amma bioenergy system

C. Chinese meridians

D. All of the above

145. The five elements of fire, earth, metal, water, and wood are associated with

A. A five-pointed star

B. Organs of the body

C. Emotions, seasons, and climates

D. All of the above

146. The primary method of water movement into and out of body compartments is
    A. Diffusion
    B. Osmosis
    C. Filtration
    D. Hydrolysis

147. The hormone that aids in determining the basal metabolic rate (BMR) is
    A. Estrogen
    B. Thyroid hormone
    C. Insulin
    D. Epinephrine

148. According to the 12 meridians, vital energy, circulation, and nutrients flow start in the
    A. Gall bladder (GB)
    B. Liver (LIV)
    C. Lung (L)
    D. Pericardium (P)

149. Which of the following is **TRUE** concerning cartilage?
    A. Except for that in the perichondrium, cartilage has no blood vessels or nerves
    B. The cells of mature cartilage are known as lacunae
    C. The resilience of cartilage is due to its collagen fiber
    D. There are three kinds of cartilage: hyaline, mosaic, and elastic

150. You have a headache and rub your temple area immediately posterior to the zygomatic part of the orbit. You are rubbing the skin, connective tissue, and muscle over which bone?
    A. Frontal
    B. Parietal
    C. Sphenoid
    D. Temporal

151. Which of the following is **TRUE** concerning the scapula?
    A. The end of the spine projects as the expanded process called the coracoid

B. The coracoid articulates with the clavicle
    C. The glenoid cavity is where the scapula and humerus articulate
    D. The lateral border of the scapula is near the vertebral column

152. For complete absorption, the average meal requires about
    A. 4 hours
    B. 10 hours
    C. 12 hours
    D. None of the above statements is accurate

153. The invisible circulation of vital energy is called
    A. Chi
    B. Regulating channel
    C. Hseuh
    D. Yin and Yang

154. The principle of a negative feedback system is
    A. To regulate hormone levels in the blood
    B. The stimuli that triggers an endocrine gland
    C. Like a thermostat in a house
    D. All of the above

155. The pancreas is an endocrine gland that secretes _____ and _____ to maintain normal blood glucose levels.
    A. Insulin and parathormone
    B. Insulin and glucagon
    C. Glucagon and pancreatic juice
    D. Insulin and progesterone

156. A synaptic transmission of a nerve impulse is
    A. A one way nerve conduction from the axon to dendrite
    B. A neurotransmitter chemical
    C. A two way nerve conduction between two axons
    D. None of these

157. An example of a neurotransmitter is
    A. Acetylcholine

B. Dopamine

C. Serotonin

D. All of these

158. A frequently used pulse point is the
    A. Jugular vein
    B. Carotid artery
    C. Popliteal artery
    D. Femoral artery

159. Which muscle tendons form the Achilles tendon?
    A. Soleus and tibialis
    B. Achilles and gastrocnemius
    C. Gastrocnemius and soleus
    D. Peroneus and soleus

160. _____ nerves regulate blood pressure.
    A. Parasympathetic
    B. Sympathetic
    C. Peripherial
    D. Cranial

161. Venous blood is found in which vessel?
    A. Pulmonary vein
    B. Pulmonary artery
    C. Aorta
    D. Arterioles

162. The kidneys are located
    A. In the GI tract
    B. Below the fifth lumbar vertebrae
    C. Opposite the twelfth thoracic vertebrae
    D. Above the liver

163. The acromion process is part of which bone?
    A. Humerus
    B. Thoracic vertebrae
    C. Clavicle
    D. Scapula

164. Manipulation of the occipital region primarily affects which meridians?
    A. BL and GB
    B. LI and SP

C. KI and TH

D. Liv and LU

165. Dorsiflexors of the ankle include
    A. Tibialis anterior
    B. Extensor digitorum and hallucis longus
    C. Peroneus
    D. All of the above

166. The deepest muscle at the back of the knee is
    A. Plantaris
    B. Popliteus
    C. Tibialis posterior
    D. Soleus

167. Medial and lateral condyles can be found on
    A. Femur and tibia
    B. Pelvis
    C. Tibia and fibula
    D. Radius and ulna

168. The olecranon process is found on the
    A. Humerus
    B. Tibia
    C. Radius
    D. Ulna

169. The obturator innervates muscles in the lower body including
    A. Gracilis
    B. Adductors
    C. Obturator externus
    D. All of the above

170. Endocrine glands
    A. Use ducts to transport their products to the site of action
    B. Include sebaceous and salivary glands
    C. Produce secretions that diffuse directly into the blood
    D. A and B

171. Chemicals that facilitate, arouse, or inhibit the transmission of nerve impulses across synapses are
    A. Hormones
    B. Histamines
    C. Steroids
    D. Neurotransmitters

172. The muscle that is responsible for the resisting or opposing action is called the
    A. Agonist or prime
    B. Synergist
    C. Antagonist
    D. Insertion

173. A sac-like membrane that contains synovial fluid and is provided around joints to prevent friction is
    A. Suture
    B. Tendon
    C. Periosteum
    D. Bursae

174. The greatest range of motion (ROM) is from
    A. Pivot joints
    B. Hinge joints
    C. Ball and socket joints
    D. Saddle joints

175. The muscle causing the desired action is the
    A. Agonist or prime mover
    B. Retinaculum
    C. Antagonist
    D. Insertion

176. The three divisions of the small intestines start to finish are
    A. Duodenum, ileum, jejunum
    B. Ascending, transverse, descending
    C. Jejunum, ileum, duodenum
    D. Duodenum, jejunum, ileum

177. The major type of muscle in the gastrointestinal (GI) tract is the
    A. Cardiac
    B. Voluntary
    C. Skeletal
    D. Smooth

178. What is the mechanical and chemical process that occurs as food is converted into an absorbable state
    A. Ingestion
    B. Digestion
    C. Homeostasis
    D. Absorption

179. The main part of the heart's conducting system is/are
    A. Sinoatrial (SA) node
    B. The atrioventricular bundle
    C. Atrioventricular (AV) node
    D. All of the above

180. Gas exchange between blood and the tissue is called
    A. Environmental respiration
    B. External respiration
    C. Internal respiration
    D. Diffusion of gas

181. The sounds created by a beating heart are due to the
    A. Contraction of the ventricles
    B. Closing of the heart valves
    C. Blood moving from one heart chamber to another
    D. Compression from the respiratory system

182. The main muscle(s) of respiration is/are
    A. Scalene
    B. Sternocleidomastoid
    C. Diaphragm
    D. Rectus abdominus

183. The main venous portal system which collects blood from the digestive organs and delivers this blood to the liver for processing, is called the
    A. Digestive portal system
    B. Intestinal portal system
    C. Gastric portal system
    D. Hepatic portal system

184. During this phase of pulmonary ventilation, air moves out of the lungs during normal _____
    A. Inhalation
    B. Exhalation
    C. Pulmonary apnea
    D. Tissue respiration

185. Which of the following is *not* one of the functions of the cardiovascular system
    A. Transportation and distribution of gases, nutrients, antibodies and hormones
    B. Protection of the body through disease fighting white blood cells
    C. Synthesis of vitamin A, D, and E
    D. Protection of the body through the clotting mechanism

186. Which of the following structures collect and filter lymph
    A. Lymph nodes
    B. Spleen
    C. Tonsils
    D. All of the above

187. The valves located between both the ventricles are the
    A. Tricuspid valves
    B. Mitral valves
    C. Sinoatrial valves
    D. A and B

188. The functional contractile unit in muscle fibers composed of actin and myosin filaments is the
    A. Sarcomere
    B. Agonist
    C. Myofibril
    D. Penniform

189. In general, where do the flexors of the wrist originate
    A. Lateral epicondyle of the humerus
    B. Greater tubercle of the humerus
    C. Medial epicondyle of the humerus
    D. Lesser tubercle of the humerus

190. Which muscle expands the thoracic cavity
    A. Internal intercostals
    B. Diaphragm
    C. Multifidus
    D. Levator scapula

ANSWERS AND RATIONALES

1.

A. The blood flow from the right atrium to the right ventricle is through the tricuspid valve to keep the blood flowing in one direction. (*Beck, p. 165*)

2.

C. The ischial tuberosity is the posterior portion of the ramus of the ischium, where the body weight is supported. (*Thompson, p. 90*)

3.

B. The Golgi tendon organ is a proprioceptor. Proprioceptors are multibranched sensory nerve endings in tendons that measure tension in the muscle. (*Beck, p. 202*)

4.

B. Adductor muscles of the upper body that bring the arms toward the body include the pectoralis major and latissimus dorsi. (*Beck, p. 126*)

5.

C. The lumbosacral plexus includes all of the spinal nerves that exit from L1 to L5 nerves supply the lower limb, not the vertebrae. (*Kapit, p. 150*)

6.

D. The 12 bilateral meridians in the body conduct energy along pathways that are related to organs and the Chi (energy). (*Tappan, p. 135*)

7.

B. Polarity therapy supports health and healing by releasing obstructions using the cradle, elbow milk, and rocking. (*Tappan, p. 210*)

8.

A. All the Yin channels meet with the deep and superficial pathways of the Conception Vessels at CV1 to CV24. (*Sohn, p. 92*)

9.

A. Sternoclavicular: The sternum of the rib cage of the axial skeleton articulates with the clavicle bone, which is part of the appendicular skeleton. (*Kapit, p. 125*)

10.

B. The pectineus, the uppermost medial thigh muscle attached to the pubis and femur, is for rotation and adduction. (*Thompson, p. 102*)

11.

B. The piriformis muscle is very close to the sciatic nerve as its origin is on the greater sciatic notch, and is innervated at L5 and S1 at the sacral plexus. (*Beck, p. 139*)

12.

C. The white blood cells (WBCs) fight any infection by engulfing and digesting bacteria and producing antibodies for protection from disease organisms. (*Beck, p. 173*)

13.

D. To practice Shiatsu well, one should begin by being in touch with the ground and make the connection to relieve tensions through breathing and increase the awareness of body weight on the floor. A feeling of support is important to convey it in our work with others. (*Lundberg, p. 28*)

14.

A. There is a force, or vibration, that, when smooth, results in good health. Techniques detect imbalance in the force and through energetic manipulation regain homeostasis. (*Sohnen-Moe, p. 62*)

15.

A. The movement of bones occurring at a synovial joint is called range of motion, and includes flexion, adduction, and rotation. (*Kapit, p. 34*)

16.

A. The Japanese word shiatsu means pressure of the fingers: shi (finger) and atsu (pressure). (*Beck, p. 567*)

17.

B. The spleen, liver, and kidney meridian pathways are all along the thigh and calf. When palming or massaging the leg with the petrissage stroke or compression all three are affected. (*Lundberg, pp. 22, 77, 100*)

18.

D. Many factors contribute to muscle fatigue, including a lactic acid buildup and depletion of oxygen, calcium, and glycogen. (*Tortora, p. 252*)

19.

D. A muscle spasm is a sudden involuntary contraction of the muscle when the nerve to the muscle is irritated. (*Beck, p. 120*)

20.

A. The first-class lever is like a seesaw as the head is resting on the vertebrae. When the head is raised the facial area is in resistance. The fulcrum is between the effort and resistance. (*Tortora, p. 271*)

21.

D. The Yin channels are located on the front of the body and the inner surfaces of the limbs and belong to the deep organs of the body, liver, spleen, and kidney. (*Lundberg, pp. 22, 77*)

22.

D. The platysma is the superficial muscle of the face that moves the lip downward and backward by inserting on the mandible. (*Tortora, p. 279*)

23.

B. The brachial plexus contributes spinal nerves through C5–C8 and T1 only. (*Tortora, p. 393*)

24.

C. The principles and techniques of Shiatsu include palming to loosen joints, thumbing for pressure and stretching and rotation to position limbs. Cross-fiber friction is used in massage for trigger points, adhesions and scar tissue. (*Lundberg, pp. 44–50*)

25.

D. The flexors at the elbow joint include the brachialis, brachioradialis, and biceps brachii. These muscles all help to flex the forearm. (*Tortora, p. 308*)

26.

A. The fascia can be manipulated through the Rolfing method. (*Beck, p. 16*)

27.

C. The pronator quadratus is responsible for pronating the forearm and wrist. (*Tortora, p. 308*)

28.

A. The hamstring muscles of the posterior thigh include the biceps femoris, semimembranosus, and semitendinosus. The adductors do not flex. (*Tortora, p. 330*)

29.

D. Four muscles form the abdominal wall, with the external oblique being the most superficial. (*Kapit, p. 43*)

30.

C. The distal phalanges are flexed by the flexor digitorum profundus. (*Thompson, p. 71*)

31.

D. When the muscles are in a stationary contraction they are in a tonic condition. (*Beck, p. 113*)

32.

D. The body has regional lymph nodes for drainage. The inguinal nodes drain the legs at the groin. (*Beck, p. 185*)

33.

A. The energy for the stomach meridian is most effective from 7 AM to 9 AM. (*Tappan, p. 173*)

34.

C. The energy for the spleen meridian is most effective from 9 AM to 11 AM. (*Tappan, p. 173*)

35.

D. PIR, RI, and PNF all are forms of MET. Postisometric relaxation is the effect of subsequent relaxation of a muscle after periods of isometric contractions. Proprioceptive neuromuscular facilitation is a variation of PIR. Reciprocal inhibition is a response of the antagonists of a muscle that has been isometrically contracted. (*Chaitow, p. 3*)

36.

C. Anatomically the structure of a bone has a membrane over the compact bone called the periosteum. (*Beck, p. 58*)

37.

B. The supinator muscle is responsible for the palm of the hand in supination. (*Thompson, p. 55*)

38.

C. A short piriformis muscle will cause the affected side to be shortened and externally rotated. Adducting the knee across the opposite ASIS will stretch the muscle. (*Chaitow, p. 83*)

39.

D. The five adductors of the hip all have their origin on the pubis to enhance hip flexion and pulling the femur closer to the midline. They include the pectineus, adductor longus, adductor brevis, adductor magnus, and the gracilis. (*Hinkle, p. 118*)

40.

D. Terminal ganglia are located at the end of an autonomic motor pathway. (*Tortora, p. 505*)

41.

B. The flow of energy for the Yin meridians is from the inferior part of the body to the superior. (*Beck, p. 564*)

42.

A. The kidney, liver, and spleen are the meridians that pass through the medial thigh area. (*Beck, p. 566*)

43.

C. The heart meridian has a point on the little finger, and energy flows from the chest to the inside of the arm. (*Tappan, p. 139*)

44.

A. The heart meridian follows the flow of blood from the chest to the arm to the end of the little finger. (*Tappan, p. 139*)

45.

D. The triple heater (warmer) is the meridian that stands for fire and has no corresponding organ along the energy path from the ring finger to the side of the head. (*Beck, p. 566*)

46.

B. The abductor muscles move an appendage away from the body. (*Beck, pp. 43, 138*)

47.

B. The vertebrae are slightly movable joints that are classified as gliding. (*Kapit, p. 33*)

48.

D. A ligament is the strong fibrous connective tissue that articulates bone to bone. (*Beck, p. 98*)

49.

D. A person who is able to receive blood from any other blood type is AB and is the universal recipient. (*Tortora, p. 585*)

50.

B. The broad surface of the radius bone is covered by a long fibrous connective tissue called the interosseous ligament. It holds the radius to the ulna and allows slight movement. (*Hinkle, p. 56*)

51.

C. The liver (LIV) meridian is located on the big toe. (*Beck, p. 566*)

52.

A. Blood returns to the heart through the hepatic portal system when digestion is completed. (*Kapit, p. 74*)

53.

C. Directional terminology is used in reference to a landmark that does not change. Two references make the statement correct; elbow is proximal (closer to head) to the hand, and the hand is distal (farther from head) to the elbow. (*Hinkle, p. 3*)

54.

A. The white matter is collectively the axons that are supported by the neuroglia cells. (*Kapit, pp. 11, 138*)

55.

C. There are approximately $5 \times 10^6/mm^3$ erythrocytes found in the blood, contributing the largest number of formed elements. (*Tortora, p. 570*)

56.

D. The kidney, spleen, and stomach are the meridians that transverse the abdomen. (*Beck, p. 566*)

57.

B. The foot is most inferior (below) to the head and not in back, in front or away from the head as the body's point of reference. (*Hinkle, p. 6*)

58.

B. The radius and proximal carpals form the radiocarpal joint (wrist). It is an ellipsoid joint that helps to pronate and supinate the forearm. (*Biel, p. 81*)

59.

A. The brachialis is an important flexor of the arm, along with the biceps brachii. (*Kapit, p. 49*)

60.
D. The medial malleolus is found on the medial side of the tibia in the leg. (*Beck, p. 95*)

61.
A. The ascending aorta gives rise to many arteries, including the left coronary artery of the heart. (*Beck, p. 166*)

62.
A. The dendrite is the structure on the neuron that carries impulses toward the cell body. (*Beck, p. 190*)

63.
B. The head of the radius articulates with the humerus at the capitulum. (*Tortora, p. 203*)

64.
C. The brachial plexus has many nerves that go into the shoulder and arm, including the median nerve. (*Kapit, p. 130*)

65.
C. The bladder meridian energy flow travels on the posterior side, starting on the head, down the back, along the leg to the toe. (*Beck, p. 566*)

66.
A. The axillary nerve is part of the brachial plexus that innervates the deltoid at the shoulder. (*Tortora, p. 340*)

67.
A. All the extensor muscles of the wrist and fingers create extension and are located between the brachioradialis and the shaft of the ulna. (*Biel, p. 97*)

68.
A. Skeletal muscle is rich in blood for quick movement, which requires ATP and gas exchange. (*Tortora, p. 257*)

69.
D. Any body temperature above 98. 6° F or 37° C is higher than normal body temperature. (*Tortora, p. 856*)

70.
C. The Yang meridian triple warmer goes from the ring finger back to the side of the head, controlling temperature, digestion, and elimination. (*Beck, p. 566*)

71.
A. The pectoralis minor and serratus anterior control abduction of the scapula. (*Beck, p. 124*)

72.
A. The 12 pairs of cranial nerves are motor or sensory, and arise from the base of the brain apart from the CNS. (*Beck, p. 191*)

73.
A. The iliac branches off the dorsal aorta to supply the legs. (*Beck, p. 175*)

74.
D. The peroneus longus is responsible for the eversion of the foot and the plantar flexion. (*Beck, p. 145*)

75.
A. The bladder meridian is massaged to affect energy as well as for sacral pain. (*Tappan, p. 140*)

76.
A. The adult normal pulse range is 70–80 beats per minute. (*Tortora, p. 645*)

77.
C. The gluteus maximus is an extender of the hip and femur. (*Beck, p. 138*)

78.
C. Blood pressure is measured in systolic and diastolic measurements. A normal systolic pressure is 120 mm/Hg and diastolic 80 mm/Hg. (*Tortora, p. 646*)

79.
A. The diaphragm is a smooth muscle in breathing and contracts during inspiration (moves down). (*Beck, p. 227*)

80.
A. Lymph fluid consists of water, cell debris, gases, metabolic waste, and bacteria. (*Beck, p. 542*)

81.
C. The flexor carpi radialis and palmaris longus are innervated by the median and the ulnar nerve and affects the flexor carpi ulnaris, flexor digitorum superficialis, and profundus. (*Biel, p. 101*)

82.
A. The medial collateral ligament is also called the tibial collateral ligament, which connects the femur to the tibia and to the medial meniscus. (*Salvo, p. 147*)

83.
C. The teres major is not part of the "SITS" muscles of the rotator cuff. It is located on the scapula and humerus for rotation and extension. (*Kapit, p. 47*)

84.
C. The nervous and endocrine systems respond to homeostatic responses. (*Tortora, p. 10*)

85.
D. Water is the most abundant inorganic molecule. (*Tortora, p. 37*)

86.
D. The pH of 6 is considered an acidic pH compared to water at 7. (*Tortora, p. 39*)

87.
D. Good body mechanics use the therapist's weight and proper postural techniques to decrease fatigue. (*Salvo, pp. 372–375*)

88.
D. The Yin of the muscle channels passes through the muscles of the forearm, arm, shoulder, and chest. (*Sohn, p. 94*)

89.
A. The horse stance or warrior stance is used to perform massage strokes that traverse short distances with both feet on the floor, toes pointing forward. (*Salvo, p. 372*)

90.
B. All the Yang channels meet with the deep and superficial pathways of the governing vessels at GV1 to GV28. (*Sohn, p. 93*)

91.
D. The outermost layer of the skin is epidermis, composed of stratified squamous epithelium. (*Tortora, p. 138*)

92.
C. One of the aging factors is a decrease in fibroblasts. (*Tortora, p. 138*)

93.
A. Ingham developed her method of Zone Therapy called reflexology and started to teach about healing the body by pressing the feet. (*Tappan, p. 234*)

94.
D. The bone matrix is hard due to the primary salt of calcium chloride. (*Tortora, p. 149*)

95.
D. Condyles are on the ends of long bones and form the joint of an articulation. (*Tortora, p. 167*)

96.
B. The cranial bones in the skull contain two paired bones: the parietal and temporal. (*Tortora, p. 173*)

97.
D. The trochlea of the humerus articulates with the ulna. (*Tortora, p. 202*)

98.
C. The medial malleolus is the ankle bone projection on the medial side. (*Tortora, p. 211*)

99.
A. The tarsal bones include the calcaneus or heel for the Achilles tendon attachment. (*Tortora, p. 212*)

100.
C. The diarthrosis joints are classified as freely movable, including the ball and socket, hinges, and pivot. (*Tortora, p. 226*)

101.
D. The thumb is classified with a saddle joint for movement at the carpal and metacarpal articulation. (*Tortora, p. 226*)

102.
D. The single hinge of the knee and elbow and the double hinge of the wrist and ankle are types of diarthroses joints. (*Tortora, p. 226*)

103.
A. The knee contains many ligaments that are intraarticular and include the ACL (anterior cruciate ligament). (*Tortora, p. 232*)

104.
D. Skeletal muscles are the only types of muscle cells that are multinucleated. (*Tortora, p. 238*)

105.
C. The Ki within the universe is used within our bodies as purification or detoxification for this energy. (*Teaguarden, p. 30*)

106.

D. Jin Shin Do developed as a preventative health art to strengthen the absorption of Ki through the techniques of acupressure, meditation, and breathing. (*Teaguarden, pp. 14, 30*)

107.

B. The lung generally is the first line of exposure and defense by a negative substance or energy and has been identified as the delicate organ. (*Sohn, pp. 110–111*)

108.

A. Atrophy is a condition in which the muscle cannot be contracted or is very weakened and begins to waste away. (*Beck, p. 123*)

109.

C. Abdominis muscle runs adjacent to the midline in a parallel direction. (*Tortora, p. 272*)

110.

A. The major cheek muscle is the buccinator, which is able to compress and blow out in the sucking motion. (*Tortora, p. 279*)

111.

B. The spinal cord in the adult ends between the first and second lumbar vertebrae, which is called conus medullaris. (*Tortora, p. 376*)

112.

A. The reflex arc does not include the brain in the rapid adjustments to homeostatic balancing. Only the spinal cord integrates the reflex action. (*Tortora, p. 384*)

113.

C. The stretch reflex is important to maintaining and adjusting muscle tone through a monosynaptic reflex arc, one motor and one sensory. (*Tortora, p. 384*)

114.

A. The axillary nerve of the brachial plexus stimulates the deltoid muscle, which is used as an injection site. (*Tortora, p. 395*)

115.

D. The sciatic nerve of the sacral plexus is composed of the common peroneal and tibial nerves arising from L4–S4. (*Tortora, p. 399*)

116.

D. The deltoid muscle of the shoulder and the supraspinatus accomplish the abduction of the humerus. (*Tortora, p. 305*)

117.

D. The adduction of the arm is accomplished by the pectoralis major of the chest, teres major, latissimus dorsi, and the coracobrachialis. (*Tortora, p. 305*)

118.

D. The erector spinae muscles are composed of three separate muscles: iliocostalis, longissimus, and spinalis. The platysma is found in the face. (*Tortora, pp. 318–321*)

119.

A. The gluteus maximus extends and rotates the thigh laterally. It does not abduct the thigh. (*Tortora, p. 323*)

120.

D. The deep muscles, including the obturator externus and internus, and piriformis accomplish lateral rotation of the thigh. (*Tortora, p. 323*)

121.

C. The sartorius muscle is the longest muscle found in the leg and laterally rotates when crossing over the knee. (*Tortora, p. 330*)

122.

A. The tendino-muscle channels are part of the full-body manipulation technique used by the Amma therapist to promote the flow of Qi, blood, and fluids. (*Sohn, p. 73*)

123.

C. The false statement is that at the chemical synapse ions do travel through gap junctions. (*Tortora, p. 364*)

124.

D. The sense of hearing is the vestibulocochlear cranial nerve—VIII. (*Tortora, p. 412*)

125.

D. The memory is associated with frontal temporal, occipital, and parietal lobe association cortex and parts of the limbic system and diencephalon. (*Tortora, p. 423*)

126.
D. The cerebral cortex has areas for muscle movement that are action-specific for motor movements. (*Tortora, p. 424*)

127.
C. Amma therapy treats the body by assessing energy imbalances and dysfunctional organs and then brings healing energy to those areas. (*Sohn, p. 6*)

128.
A. The hypothalamus part of the brain regulates the balance of sympathetic and parasympathetic activity. (*Tortora, p. 513*)

129.
B. The liver and spleen meridians are stimulated when the dorsum of the foot is massaged. (*Beck, p. 566*)

130.
B. The hormone glucagon stimulates formation of glucose from lactate and amino acids. (*Tortora, p. 549*)

131.
D. Some hormones are known by alternate names, including vasopressin for antidiuretic hormone (ADH). (*Tortora, p. 534*)

132.
A. There is no blood pressure in the veins as compared to the arteries. (*Beck, p. 168*)

133.
C. The liquid portion of the blood is plasma, which is 55% of the total volume. (*Tortora, p. 568*)

134.
D. The blood is the transport system for metabolic wastes, gases, nutrients, hormones, and salts. (*Tortora, p. 567*)

135.
C. The mediastinum is the medial part of the thoracic cavity containing the heart. (*Tortora, p. 592*)

136.
C. Ganglia are masses of neurons that extend along the outside of the spine and synapse with other neurons. (*Beck, p. 196*)

137.
C. In blood flow, the lungs return oxygenated blood to the left side of the heart at the atrium. (*Tortora, p. 673*)

138.
D. The aorta artery branches after it leaves the heart with the major brachiocephalic. (*Tortora, p. 648*)

139.
B. The vena cava branches into the jugular vein, which drains the blood from the brain. (*Tortora, p. 663*)

140.
D. Drainage of lymph from the right leg enters the cisterna chyli and then the left thoracic duct. (*Tortora, p. 686*)

141.
D. To follow the Yin-Yang principle is to change from season to season, light to dark, warm to cold, and follow the continual rhythm of all life. (*Teaguarden, p. 23*)

142.
D. An aerobic process converts glucose into pyruvic acid, provided a blood supply and oxygen are available. (*Tortora, p. 826*)

143.
D. Iron is a mineral that is part of the hemoglobin in the RBC. (*Tortora, p. 848*)

144.
B. The Amma bioenergy system is a series of complex channels throughout the body and organs. (*Sohn, p. 70*)

145.
D. The heart, spleen, lung, kidney, and liver, as well as the seasons, the climate, and emotions are all associated with the five-pointed star of the elements. (*Sohn, p. 21*)

146.
B. The diffusion of water is called osmosis. A concentration gradient difference forces this function. (*Tortora, p. 905*)

147.

B. The thyroid gland secretes the thyroid hormone, which aids in determining the basal metabolic rate (BMR). (*Tortora, p. 855*)

148.

C. The lung (L) meridian is the one with the most vital energy. (*Tappan, p. 135*)

149.

A. Cartilage is a connective tissue that has few or no blood vessels or nerves. (*Tortora, p. 110*)

150.

C. The sphenoid bone is the keystone of the cranial floor because it articulates with many bones and is a common area for a headache massage. (*Tortora, p. 176*)

151.

C. The glenoid cavity is where the scapula and humerus articulate. (*Tortora, p. 200*)

152.

A. In about a four-hour period, a meal has been completely digested. (*Tortora, p. 844*)

153.

A. The Chi is the Chinese word for the energy flow of the meridian. (*Tappan, p. 136*)

154.

D. The endocrine system functions as a negative feedback system by regulating the hormone levels in the blood. When the blood level reaches normal, the target organ is stimulated to stop secreting, i.e, negative feedback to the gland. (*Salvo, p. 267*)

155.

B. Insulin decreases blood glucose and glucagon increases blood glucose levels. The alpha cells of the pancreas secrete both. (*Salvo, p. 271*)

156.

A. A synaptic transmission is one electrochemical method by which the nerve impulse from one axon bridges the synaptic gap (synaptic cleft) to the nerve derdrite of the next neuron. (*Salvo, p. 237*)

157.

D. There are 30 known neurotransmitters in the body that facilitate, arouse, or inhibit the transmission of nerve impulses between synapses. They include acetylcholine, serotonin, dopamine, epinephrine, histamine, and more. (*Salvo, p. 238*)

158.

B. The carotid artery is used frequently for pulse since it is easy to record on the neck area even if a person is dressed. There is no pulse in a vein. (*Salvo, p. 287*)

159.

C. The insertion of the soleus and gastrocnemius muscle is the Achilles tendon on the posterior surface of the calcaneus. (*Fritz, Paholsky, & Grosenbach, p. 374*)

160.

B. The sympathetic nervous system regulates the blood pressure to the arterioles. As the vessels become more remote from the heart, the pressure decreases. (*Fritz, Paholsky, & Grosenbach, p. 475*)

161.

B. The pulmonary artery carries carbon dioxide from the right ventricle to the lungs for gas exchange. It is the only artery that transports oxygen poor blood away from the heart. (*Fritz, Paholsky, & Grosenbach, p. 469*)

162.

C. The kidneys are a pair of organs located bilaterally in the upper lumbar region opposite the twelfth thoracic vertebrae. (*Salvo, p. 336*)

163.

D. The acromion process is found on the lateral end of the spine of the scapula and forms the top of the shoulder and articulates with the clavicle with the acromioclavicular ligament. (*Fritz, Paholsky, & Grosenbach, p. 274*)

164.

A. The bladder and gall bladder are Yang channels that flow down the back of the head and neck and are the two pathways affected by occipital pressure. (*Lundberg, pp. 76, 110*)

165.

D. The tibialis, extensor digitorum, and hallucis and peroneus tertius perform the dorsiflexion of the ankle. (*Sieg and Adams, p. 124*)

166.

B. The popliteus muscle initiates knee flexion and is the deepest at the posterior of the knee. (*Sieg and Adams, p. 104*)

167.

A. The femur and the tibia each have a medial and lateral condyle, which serve for muscle attachment. (*Sieg and Adams, p. 81*)

168.

D. The olecranon process is at the elbow joint located on the proximal end of the ulna. (*Sieg and Adams, p. 7*)

169.

D. The obturator innervates the gracilis, adductors, and obturator externus of the thigh. (*Sieg and Adams, p. 127*)

170.

C. Endocrine glands secrete hormones directly into the blood stream; they are also called "ductless glands." (*Salvo, p. 266*)

171.

D. Neurotransmitters are the ninety-nine percent chemical cause of neural impulses that are facilitators across the synaptic cleft. (*Salvo, p. 238*)

172.

C. The antagonist or opposing muscle must resist, or yield to the joint motion initiated by the agonist. (*Salvo, p. 164*)

173.

D. The bursae provide cushion and prevent rubbing of tendon during muscle contraction. They contain the synovial membrane that secretes synovial fluid for lubrication of joints. (*Salvo, p. 112*)

174.

C. The ball and socket joint or sphenoid, triaxial joint has the greatest range of motion like in the hip and shoulder. (*Salvo, p. 116*)

175.

A. The agonist or prime mover, is the muscle most responsible for causing the desired joint action. (*Salvo, p. 164*)

176.

D. The small intestine has three divisions starting with the 10–12 inch duodcnum, the intermediate section is the 6 foot jejunum, and ends with the 9 foot ileum. (*Salvo, p. 322*)

177.

D. The gastrointestinal tract is made up of the involuntary smooth muscle that starts in the esophagus, stomach, small intestine and ends with the large intestine. (*Salvo, p. 319*)

178.

B. Digestion occurs through chewing, peristalsis and chemical enzymes, and hydrolysis to prepare the food ingested for absorption. (*Salvo, p. 318*)

179.

D. The sinoatrial (SA) node, atrioventricular (AV) node and atrioventricular bundle are all part of the conduction system of the heart, which are made up of modified cardiac cells. (*Salvo, p. 284*)

180.

C. Internal respiration or tissue respiration is the diffusion of oxygen from the blood capillaries to the tissue cells. (*Salvo, p. 309*)

181.

B. The sounds by a beating heart are due to the closing of the hearts valves: tricuspid and bicuspid, pulmonary and aortic. (*Salvo, p. 285*)

182.

C. The muscle of respiration is the diaphragm, a dome-shaped muscular partition that separates the thoracic cavity from the abdominal cavity. (*Salvo, p. 306*)

183.

D. The hepatic portal system collects blood from the digestive system to be processed before it enters the systemic circulation. (*Salvo, p. 289*)

184.

B. During normal exhalation of pulmonary ventilation, the air is forced out of the lungs as the diaphragm relaxes. (*Salvo, p. 307*)

185.

C. The synthesis of Vitamin A, D, and E is not a function of the cardiovascular system. It only produces clotting proteins and blood cells in the bone marrow. (*Salvo, p. 278*)

186.

A. The lymph flows into the afferent vessels and leaves through the efferent vessels of the lymph nodes. (*Salvo, p. 294*)

187.

D. The heart valves that separate the atria from the ventricles are called tricuspid on the right side and mitral (or bicuspid) on the left side. (*Salvo, p. 284*)

188.

A. The sarcomere is the microscopic contractile unit of the myofibril. It contains two predominant proteins called actin and myosin that move across according to the sliding filament theory of muscle contraction. (*Salvo, p. 158*)

189.

C. The flexors of the forearm have their origin on the medial epicondyle of the humerus and insert on the metacarpals. (*Salvo, p. 183*)

190.

B. The diaphragm is the breathing muscle that expands the thoracic cavity during inhalation. (*Salvo, p. 223*)

2 Clinical Pathology and Recognition of Various Conditions

OBJECTIVES: Major areas of knowledge/content included in this chapter are based on the NCTMB exam topics and percentage of questions (20%)

1. History and client intake process
   - Impact of client medical history on disease and recovery
   - History of abuse and trauma related to disease and recovery
   - Emotional states and stress leading to disease
   - Effects of life stages on basic health and well-being

2. Disease and injury-related conditions
   - Signs and symptoms of disease
   - Indications and contraindications
   - Physiological changes and healing mechanisms

1. Which muscle would be paralyzed if the sciatic nerve were severed?
   A. Trapezius
   B. Biceps femoris
   C. Gluteus maximus
   D. Erector spinae

2. Senile lentigo or liver spots on the skin
   A. Are not contraindicated for massage
   B. Are contraindicated for massage
   C. Should be referred to a dermatologist
   D. Can be a symptom of cancer

3. If massage is used in early stages of fracture healing, it should be given particularly on the area
   A. Proximal to the actual site
   B. Distal to the actual site
   C. Medial to the actual site
   D. Lateral to the actual site

4. Contraindicated fungal skin infections include
   A. Herpes simplex
   B. Warts
   C. Athletes foot
   D. All of the above

5. Which condition is present when there is an injury of the ulnar nerve at the elbow?
   A. Inability to flex fingers fully
   B. Spasticity
   C. Flaccidity
   D. Spasms

6. In treating a patient with kyphosis, which muscle or muscles should the massage therapist try to stretch and relax?
   A. Pectorals
   B. Rhomboids
   C. Erector spinae
   D. Trapezius

7. If a client has skin damaged by the burns of fire, chemicals or radiation and require grafting
   A. Massage can be done after the graft heals
   B. This is a third degree burn
   C. Gentle range of motion (ROM) can increase mobility
   D. All of the above

8. Which technique is recommended for rheumatoid arthritis?
   A. Effleurage
   B. Gentle friction
   C. Kneading
   D. Tapotement

9. Massage can be beneficial for a headache with symptom(s) of
   A. Sinus pressure
   B. Vascular disruption
   C. Release of toxins
   D. All of the above

10. Thorough assessment of a client's medical intake reveals
    A. Addictions
    B. Emotional problems
    C. Personal information
    D. Contraindications for massage

11. Herpes Simplex is a _____ infection of the skin.
    A. Bacterial
    B. Viral
    C. Non-contagious
    D. Autoimmune

12. Adhesion development and excessive scarring following trauma can be prevented or reduced with
    A. Joint movements
    B. Petrissage
    C. Friction massage
    D. Passive movements

13. Most muscle strains occur on the
_____.
    A. Tendon
    B. Antagonist muscle
    C. Tight, spasmed muscle
    D. All of the above

14. Techniques to avoid using on a pregnant client are heavy percussion and
    A. Deep tissue massage
    B. Tapotement
    C. Petrissage
    D. Lymph stimulation

15. Which of the following is a virus-induced mass produced by uncontrolled epithelial skin cell growth?
    A. Contusion
    B. Cyst
    C. Laceration
    D. Wart

16. If a client has a hernia, the best approach is
    A. A referral to physician
    B. Local contraindication around affected area
    C. To reschedule appointment
    D. Start the massage in a prone position

17. In order to evaluate projected pain it is necessary to know the
    A. Portion of the brain involved
    B. Proximal nerve that is compressed
    C. Distal nerve that is compressed
    D. None of the above

18. When a client has fibromyalgia it is best to
    A. Avoid giving a massage due to the pain
    B. Assess the "tender points" and tailor the treatment
    C. Wait until the disease is in remission
    D. Refer to a reflexologist

19. A sprain with extensive swelling is caused by an injury to the
    A. Muscle
    B. Wrist
    C. Ligament
    D. Tendon

20. Massage can be beneficial if a client is recovering from pneumonia because
    A. Tapotement and vibration on the chest can help drain the secretions
    B. The client is no longer contagious
    C. The client can cough up phlegm
    D. None of the above

21. Injuries that have a gradual onset or reoccur often are called
    A. Sprains
    B. Occupational
    C. Acute
    D. Chronic

22. The disease(s) of the nervous system that is (are) contraindicated to massage is (are)
    A. Multiple sclerosis
    B. Meningitis
    C. Sciatica
    D. Parkinson's disease

23. A muscle strain that involves a partial tear of 10% to 50% of the muscle fibers is classified as
    A. Grade I
    B. Grade II
    C. Grade III
    D. Parietal

24. Which nerve is affected in carpal tunnel syndrome?
    A. Axillary
    B. Median
    C. Medial pectoral
    D. Radial

25. The popliteal fossa is an endangerment site because of the
    A. Lymph nodes
    B. Tibial and peroneal nerves
    C. Median cubital vein
    D. Kidney

26. What client information is critical in the history intake process
    A. Previous surgeries
    B. Illnesses
    C. Medical conditions
    D. All of the above

27. To reduce adhesions and fibrosis, which of the following movements is used?
    A. Cross-fiber friction
    B. Wringing
    C. Pressing
    D. Squeezing

28. Massage interfaces with the effects of many medications and therefore it is important to reference drugs in the (a)
    A. *Gray's Anatomy*
    B. *Physicians' Desk Reference*
    C. *Webster's dictionary*
    D. Medical dictionary

29. Massage therapists should be able to assess the effects of medications that alter muscle tone, cardiovascular function, as well as
    A. Anticoagulants
    B. Personality
    C. Analgesics
    D. All of the above

30. Why is it important to have the illnesses and/or medical conditions available before a massage?
    A. The state requires this
    B. For the purpose of assessing any potential contraindication

C. If you are giving a relaxation massage, it is not necessary
D. It is not necessary to do an intake unless you are a nurse

31. Pathogenic organisms cause the development of many disease processes and include
    A. Virus and bacteria
    B. Fungi
    C. Protozoa
    D. All of the above

32. Severe strain of the trapezius and deltoid muscles is called
    A. Racquetball shoulder
    B. Tennis elbow
    C. Skier's snap
    D. Bowler's break

33. Overstretching of the gracilis and adductor muscle on the inner thigh results from
    A. Soccer
    B. Tennis
    C. Horseback riding
    D. Bowling

34. The client may react to pain with
    A. Fear and anxiety
    B. Ischemic response
    C. Active movement
    D. Passive movement

35. Severe varicose veins are a (an) _____ for massage.
    A. Indication
    B. Taboo
    C. Embolus
    D. Contraindication

36. Sciatic nerve damage diminishes ability to
    A. Flex the hip
    B. Flex the knee
    C. Adduct the hip
    D. Abduct the hip

37. Swelling of one entire leg is usually caused by pathology in
    A. Heart muscle
    B. A blood vessel
    C. Kidney
    D. Liver

38. In a patient with subdeltoid bursitis, the pain is worse if the arm is
    A. Abducted
    B. Adducted
    C. Hyperextended
    D. Laterally rotated

39. Arthritis is a (an)
    A. Vitamin D deficiency
    B. Vitamin C deficiency
    C. Inflammation of the joints
    D. Bone fracture

40. Facial paralysis can be due to a lesion in which cranial nerve?
    A. III
    B. VI
    C. VII
    D. VIII

41. In chronic swelling around the patella, what massage technique do you use on the thigh?
    A. Kneading of the thigh
    B. Friction of the knee
    C. Effleurage proximal to knee
    D. Effleurage distal to knee

42. Inflammation of the walls of the vein is called
    A. Aneurysm
    B. Phlebitis
    C. Varicose vein
    D. Atherosclerosis

43. When treating swelling due to a dislocated knee, which technique is valuable?
    A. Effleurage
    B. Kneading
    C. Tapotement
    D. Friction

44. Most stress and pain patterns that respond to therapeutic massage involve the
    A. Circulatory and nervous system
    B. Nervous and endocrine systems
    C. Muscle system
    D. None of the above

45. To treat the seventh cranial palsy (Bell's palsy), brisk friction kneading should be done
    A. From the mandible to hairline vertically
    B. From the hairline to maxilla
    C. Transversely with both hands
    D. Not at all

46. According to Cyriax, which stroke is **BEST** for tenosynovitis?
    A. Effleurage
    B. Transverse friction
    C. Percussion
    D. Vibration

47. Muscular dystrophy is characterized by degeneration and wasting of
    A. Muscle tissue
    B. Nervous tissue
    C. Epithelial tissue
    D. All of the above

48. Massage is helpful with medical supervision for
    A. Rheumatoid arthritis
    B. Lupus
    C. Ankylosing spondylitis
    D. All of the above

49. A term that means an abnormally low level of WBCs is
    A. Leukopenia
    B. Leukocytopenia
    C. Leukocytosis
    D. Leukophoma

50. Tight hamstrings contribute to back pain due to
   A. Limited lumbar movement
   B. Ischial origin
   C. Limited hip flexion
   D. All of the above

51. Carpal tunnel syndrome affects the
   A. Volar aspect of the wrist
   B. Dorsal wrist
   C. Anterior forearm
   D. Forearm extensors

52. When there is damage to the ulnar nerve with the inability to flex the fingers strongly, which condition would be present?
   A. Flaccidity
   B. Spasticity
   C. Spasm
   D. All of the above

53. Cutting the median nerve results in the inability to
   A. Flex the thumb
   B. Extend the wrist
   C. Extend the elbow
   D. Supinate the arm

54. Which is an example of a fungus infection?
   A. Athlete's foot
   B. Furuncle
   C. Typhoid
   D. Dysentery

55. Fusiform swelling in the fingers and joint calcification of the hand are seen in
   A. Gout
   B. Arthritis
   C. Polio
   D. Rheumatoid arthritis

56. Loss of function of the wrist and outer fingers is due to an injury to the
   A. Brachial plexus
   B. Radial nerve
   C. Median nerve
   D. Ulnar nerve

57. A survivor of abuse can benefit from massage by
   A. Feeling a sense of safeness
   B. Releasing or letting go some of the abuse
   C. Retrieving memory
   D. All of the above

58. Sciatic nerve injury may have symptoms of
   A. A herniated disc
   B. A dislocated hip
   C. Osteoarthritis of the lumbosacral spine
   D. All of the above

59. Shin splint syndrome affects the
   A. Lateral malleolus
   B. Periosteum around the tibia
   C. Fibula
   D. All of the above

60. Our emotions can lead to disease with the excess use of
   A. Food
   B. Nicotine
   C. Alcohol and drugs
   D. All of the above

61. Somatic pain arises from stimulation of
   A. Organ receptors
   B. Noxious material
   C. Receptors of the skin, muscles, or joints
   D. Referred areas

62. In pregnancy a contraindication for prenatal massage is
   A. Varicose veins
   B. Toxemia
   C. Dizziness
   D. All of the above

63. The following deviations that suggest the need for evaluation and referral for cardio-vascular clients are
    A. Pulse over 90 or under 60
    B. Red, warm, or hard veins
    C. Pain and tenderness of extremities
    D. All of the above

64. Flaccid paralysis can be benefited by the
    A. Decrease in metabolic heat production
    B. Increase in heart rate and blood pressure
    C. Deep stroking and kneading massage
    D. Relaxation of muscle tissue

65. Myofascial pain syndrome is also known as
    A. Myofascitis
    B. Fibromyositis
    C. Myofascitis trigger points
    D. All of the above

66. Pain sensations are modified by the release of neurochemicals from the CNS, including
    A. Adrenalin
    B. Endorphins and enkephalins
    C. Thyroxin
    D. Prostaglandins

67. Massage therapy is used for pain control in
    A. Labor and delivery
    B. Neuritis, neuralgia
    C. Whiplash
    D. All of the above

68. A systemic inflammatory disease is a chronic condition such as
    A. Arthritis
    B. Bronchitis
    C. Asthma
    D. All of the above

69. The intake history of a client suffering from childhood abuse is very important because
    A. You can act as a psychotherapist

B. It defines client boundaries and assures protection
    C. It is easy for a client to receive a massage
    D. You will be able to make a diagnosis

70. A massage therapist needs to know that the mechanism of pain includes
    A. Physiological aspects
    B. Social aspects
    C. Psychological aspects
    D. All of the above

71. A first-degree burn is characterized by
    A. Involvement of the dermis and epidermis
    B. Blisters
    C. Severe pain
    D. A typical sunburn

72. A second-degree burn is characterized by
    A. Involvement of the entire epidermis and possibly some of the dermis
    B. No loss of skin functions
    C. Damage to most hair follicles and sweat glands
    D. Never scarring

73. What is the name of the fracture of the distal end of the radius in which the distal fragment is displaced posteriorly?
    A. Stress fracture
    B. Spiral fracture
    C. Pott's fracture
    D. Colles' fracture

74. Which of the following is defined as the degeneration of cartilage allowing the bony ends to touch, and usually associated with the elderly?
    A. Osteoarthritis
    B. Osteogenic sarcoma
    C. Osteomyelitis
    D. Osteopenia

75. Limitation due to the stretching of fibrous tissues is called
    A. Hard end feel
    B. Springy end feel
    C. Soft end feel
    D. Acute inflammation

76. Which ligament is stretched or torn in about 70% of all serious knee injuries?
    A. Anterior cruciate
    B. Arculate popliteal
    C. Lateral collateral
    D. Medial collateral

77. When injured by trauma or infection, neurons of the central nervous system
    A. Repair slowly
    B. Don't repair
    C. Require transplants
    D. Self-destruct

78. A condition of the skin marked by elevations with clear fluid from contact with poison ivy is called a
    A. Cyst
    B. Vesicle
    C. Macule
    D. Laceration

79. Cancer is a disease that can be spread through the
    A. Genes
    B. Lymphatic and blood system
    C. Endocrine system
    D. Digestive system

80. Weak thumb movements, pain in the palm and fingers, and an inability to pronate the forearm is characteristic of an injury to which nerve?
    A. Median
    B. Medial pectoral
    C. Musculocutaneous

D. Radial

81. Massage is **NOT** performed on an area that is
    A. Bleeding
    B. Swollen
    C. Burned
    D. All of the above

82. Local anesthetics, such as procaine (Novacain), block pain and other sensations by
    A. Distracting the signal to the brain
    B. Numbing the blood vessels next to the cut
    C. Preventing the voltage leakage channels from leaking
    D. Preventing the opening of voltage-gated sodium channels

83. Epilepsy is characterized by
    A. Short, recurrent periodic attacks of motor, sensory, or psychological malfunction
    B. Epileptic seizures, which are initiated by abnormal, synchronous electrical discharges from the brain
    C. A person often contracting skeletal muscles involuntarily
    D. All of the above

84. Which of the following is **TRUE** about headaches?
    A. Analgesic and tranquilizing compounds are generally not effective for migraine headaches
    B. Migraines have been found to be helped by drugs that constrict the blood vessels
    C. Tension headaches classically occur in the occipital and temporal muscles
    D. All of the above

85. Loss of function of an entire arm is due to injury of the
    A. Ulnar nerve

B. Median nerve

C. Radial nerve

D. Brachial plexus

86. A ringing, roaring, or clicking in the ears is known as
    A. Keratitis
    B. Mydriasis
    C. Scotoma
    D. Tinnitus

87. A lower-than-normal number of RBCs is termed
    A. Hypoxia
    B. Erythropoietin
    C. Normoblastin
    D. Anemia

88. A rapid resting heart or pulse rate over 100 beats per minute is termed
    A. Bradycardia
    B. Myocardia
    C. Pericardia
    D. Tachycardia

89. The artificial cleansing and excretion of waste products from the blood is properly termed
    A. Hemodialysis
    B. Blood clearance
    C. Kidney evacuation
    D. Membrane indwelling

90. Cardiac conditions, diabetes, lung disease, and high or low blood pressure are examples of contraindications for
    A. Hydrotherapy
    B. Complications
    C. Side effects
    D. Benefits

91. Dysfunction caused by physical trauma or strain is associated with the
    A. Autonomic nervous system
    B. Sympathetic nervous system

C. Pain-spasm-pain cycle

D. Parasympathetic nervous system

92. Which of the following causes an increase in body temperature?
    A. Thyroid hormones
    B. Increased body production of epinephrine and norepinephrine into the blood
    C. Skeletal muscles contraction
    D. All of the above

93. Acquired immune deficiency syndrome (AIDS) is caused by HIV, which is an acronym for
    A. Having the immune virus
    B. Hapten immune virus
    C. Hepatic immune virus
    D. Human immunodeficiency virus

94. Which term means an exaggeration of the lumbar curve of the vertebral column?
    A. Lordosis
    B. Kyphosis
    C. Scoliosis
    D. Spina bifida

95. The symptoms of an upper respiratory infection including bronchitis, cold, and sinusitis can benefit from
    A. Light massage to area
    B. Tapotement on the chest
    C. Friction to the pectoral muscles
    D. Slapping on the back

96. A chronic, inflammatory disorder that produces sporadic narrowing of airways with periods of coughing, difficult breathing and wheezing is called
    A. Asthma
    B. Bronchitis
    C. Emphysema
    D. Tuberculosis

97. All of the following are local (regional) contraindications for massage **EXCEPT**
    A. Recent burn
    B. Undiagnosed lump
    C. Open sore
    D. Shock

98. Somatic pain arises from stimulation of receptors in the skin or from stimulation of receptors in the
    A. Viscera
    B. Peritoneum
    C. Brain
    D. Muscle, joints, tendons, and fascia

99. Acute inflammation is a massage
    A. Side effect
    B. Contraindication
    C. Indication
    D. Benefit

100. Dr. Travell and Dr. Chaitow agree that gentle stretching to reset the normal resting length of the muscle must follow therapy using
    A. Polarity
    B. Kinesiology
    C. Trigger points
    D. Meridians

101. In difficult joint movement, the main objective is
    A. Active assistive joint movement
    B. Passive joint movements
    C. Active resistive joint movement
    D. Range of motion (ROM)

102. In runner's cramp, the massage treatment is
    A. Ice application
    B. Compression on stress points
    C. Cross-fiber friction and shaking calf
    D. All of the above

103. Skin conditions contraindicate massage because
    A. They might be contagious to the practitioner
    B. Of interference with the massage
    C. Of medication and bandages
    D. The client has an infection

104. Psoriasis, a chronic skin disease
    A. Is scaly with pink, itchy patches, but not contagious
    B. Is not contraindicated
    C. Is locally contraindicated in the acute stage
    D. All of the above

105. Massage is contraindicated for the following skin disorders
    A. Incision
    B. Wound related to diabetes
    C. Bedsores
    D. All of the above

106. Gout is a disease that
    A. Is an inflammatory arthritis caused by uric acid around the joint
    B. Affects the liver and pancreas
    C. Is completely contraindicated
    D. Cannot be corrected by diet

107. In the first trimester of pregnancy
    A. Any massage is contraindicated
    B. Deep abdominal work is contraindicated
    C. All prenatal massage is indicated
    D. Massage therapist needs a referral from an orthopedist

108. Breast cancer and massage therapy of the breast
    A. Are still considered untouchable
    B. Have shown to be beneficial in some cases

C. Should not be attempted to prevent metastasis

D. None of the above

109. A client who reports hepatitis on the medical history
   A. Can be contagious and should avoid massage
   B. Has an inflammation of the liver
   C. Must be cleared by a physician for massage
   D. All of the above

110. Diverticulitis can be defined as
   A. Colon cancer
   B. A hernia in the esophagus
   C. Small pouches that protrude from the colon
   D. Polyps in the sigmoid colon

111. Massage is indicated in subacute
   A. Common cold
   B. Influenza
   C. Pneumonia
   D. All of the above

112. In the case of a client with HIV/AIDS
   A. Massage is indicated
   B. Massage is contraindicated
   C. The massage therapist must wear latex gloves
   D. A massage is only indicated in the final stages

113. Paths of infection of a pathogen include
   A. Pathogen transmission by broken skin
   B. Pathogen transmission by inhalation
   C. Pathogen transmission by contact of mucous membrane
   D. All of the above

114. When should the massage therapist use gloves?
   A. If the therapist has a break in the skin
   B. If the client request the use of gloves
   C. Internal TMJ
   D. All of the above

115. Which of the following medical condition(s) would be contraindicated
   A. Scoliosis
   B. Contact lenses
   C. Arthritis
   D. None of the above

116. The most important risk factors of cancer are
   A. Genetic predisposition and age
   B. Hormonal factors and sex
   C. Diet and exercise
   D. A and B

117. Palpatory assessment of body temperature is significant
   A. To detect decreased circulation in toes and fingers
   B. To detect fever/infection or inflammation
   C. To warn of restriction in tissues
   D. All of the above

118. A gait assessment of a clients walking pattern can detect
   A. Areas of posture imbalance
   B. Areas of pain
   C. Flat feet
   D. A and B

119. If a client indicates hypoglycemia on the medical intake
   A. Massage is contraindicated
   B. Deep muscle treatment is important for better circulation
   C. Massage is fine but the client should eat after massage
   D. Refer them for a glucose test

120. If a client indicates diabetes mellitus on the medical intake
    A. Massage is contraindicated
    B. A massage should only be given by a nurse or medical practitioner
    C. A relaxing and gentle massage is indicated
    D. Be sure they drink 8 glasses of water before getting a massage

121. If a client has emphysema the muscles to address include
    A. Deltoid and trapezius
    B. Sternocleidomastoid, scalenes, and pectoralis minor
    C. Erector spinae and rhomboids
    D. Diaphragm and pectoralis major

Answers and Rationales

1.
B. The biceps femoris would be paralyzed if the sciatic nerve were severed, since it controls the flexion of the posterior thigh and leg. *(Beck, p. 210; Kapit, p. 149)*

2.
A. Massage is fine for clients with liver or age spots. They are only brown patches of skin in older people due to excessive sun exposure. *(Salvo, p. 93)*

3.
A. Massage to the proximal area of a fracture promotes healing by stimulating circulation. *(Beck, p. 99)*

4.
C. Athletes foot is a fungal skin infection that has rings of red tissue and can bleed, break, and ooze. Local massage is contraindicated because the infection is contagious. *(Salvo, p. 94)*

5.
C. The sensation and motion that is eliminated from the elbow to the fingers due to nerve damage as called flaccidity. *(Beck, p. 209)*

6.
A. Massage to the pectorals of the chest, by stretching and relaxing, can aid the exaggerated convex curve of the thoracic spine. *(Beck, p. 102)*

7.
D. Massage should be done when skin is healed or grafts are healed. Massage and range of motion are indicated to increase circulation and prevent adhesions from forming. *(Salvo, p. 95)*

8.
B. Gentle friction helps to milk out body fluids from the inflamed joint. It also softens the massed ground substance between layers of tissue. *(Beck, pp. 100, 318)*

9.
D. Massage can benefit a pain or dull ache in the head or neck causing sinus pressure, muscle tension, release of toxins, or vascular disruption. *(Fritz, p. 402)*

10.
D. Contraindications should be revealed when the client's history is taken. They can include past/present diseases, disorders, and psychological problems. *(Beck, pp. 253–259)*

11.
B. Herpes simplex or fever blister is a viral infection that lies dormant and appears when there are stimuli such as radiation, hormonal changes or emotional upset. *(Salvo, p. 94)*

12.
C. Adhesions and scarring can be relieved by regular friction massage. Constrictions can be reduced as the muscle tissue heals. *(Beck, p. 253)*

13.
D. Muscle strains are the injury of a muscle or tendon due to a violent contraction, forced stretching or spasm of the antagonistic muscle, which is the one that resists the creating of the action. *(Salvo, p. 166)*

14.
A. Massage during pregnancy should be soothing and relaxing, never deep tissue massage or abdominal kneading or deep abdominal massage. *(Beck, p. 260)*

15.
D. Warts are known to be caused by viruses causing the skin to grow in an uncontrolled fashion. *(Tortora, p. 142)*

16.
B. Local massage is contraindicated; general massage is fine unless client is in pain. *(Salvo, p. 167)*

17.
B. Pain is perceived in the tissue supplied by the proximal nerve to the location. *(Fritz, p. 93)*

18.
B. Fibromyalgia is a myofascial syndrome, which is a chronic inflammatory disease that affects muscle and related connective tissue. It is best to assess the condition and trigger points before giving a massage. *(Salvo, p. 166)*

19.

C. An injury to a joint with a tearing or stretching of the ligament and swelling is considered a severe sprain. *(Beck, p. 100)*

20.

A. Tapotement and vibration on the chest help to drain the secretions that build up in the alveoli. The exudates are substances that have been slowly discharged from the cells as waste products. *(Salvo, p. 312)*

21.

D. Chronic injuries occur over time or are long lasting, and can benefit from gentle massage depending on the injury. *(Beck, p. 508)*

22.

B. Meningitis is contraindicated to massage because it is an infection and inflammation of the meninges that causes severe headaches, vertigo, elevated temperature, pulse, and respiration. *(Salvo, p. 257)*

23.

B. Grade II muscle strain has pain and some loss of function and some tissue bleeding. *(Beck, p. 120)*

24.

B. The median nerve of the brachial plexus is injured in carpal tunnel syndrome by the compression of the nerve through the carpal tunnel. *(Tortora, p. 394)*

25.

B. Endangerment sites on the body represent areas that can be injured due to exposure of vessels, organs, and nerves to deep massage. The tibial and peroneal nerve are endangered in the fossa of the knee. *(Beck, p. 265)*

26.

D. It is important in the assessment of a new client that all medical history, physical and emotional is considered before the first massage session. *(Salvo, p. 454)*

27.

A. Cross-fiber friction is the best stroke to prevent or reduce adhesions, and fibrosis manipulation moves fibers apart from each other. *(Beck, p. 557)*

28.

B. The *Physicians' Desk Reference* helps therapists to recognize the indications and contraindications to a client's medication. *(Fritz, p. 99)*

29.

D. Because many medications have side effects, it is important to be familiar with the various types that affect different areas of the body and mind. *(Fritz, p. 99)*

30.

B. It is important to do an assessment of the medical conditions and illnesses so that the practitioner is aware of any contraindication. *(Salvo, p. 454)*

31.

D. Many viruses, bacteria, protozoa, and worms cause pathogenic diseases, which must be prevented by use of sanitary conditions and are contraindicated for massage. *(Fritz, p. 109)*

32.

A. The shoulder and back muscles can be strained from sports such as racquetball and tennis. *(Beck, p. 532)*

33.

C. The gracilis and adductor muscles are stretched by the action of horseback riding. *(Thompson, p. 109)*

34.

A. Depending on the level of pain and experience related to an injury, a client's fear and anxiety can vary. *(Beck, p. 38)*

35.

D. If a client has varicose veins, it is not recommended to apply massage. This is a contraindication. *(Beck, pp. 256–257)*

36.

B. The sciatic nerve innervates the leg, and damage can limit the mobility of knee flexing. *(Beck, pp. 110, 142)*

37.

B. Edema, or swelling, can result from phlebitis, a blockage in the venous system. *(Beck, p. 170)*

38.

A. Joint mobility, especially abduction, is limited at the bursae due to trauma or repeated irritation. *(Beck, p. 101)*

39.

C. An inflammatory condition of the joints and bone damage is characteristic of arthritis. *(Beck, p. 101)*

40.

C. The nerve that controls facial muscles is number VII and would affect any facial paralysis. *(Beck, p. 195)*

41.

C. Effleurage is the best massage technique for moving fluid from the knee and back to the heart and lymphatic ducts. *(Tappan, p. 102)*

42.

B. Pain, swelling, and inflammation are characteristic of phlebitis of the veins. *(Beck, p. 256)*

43.

A. Effleurage around swelling is advantageous for knee injuries. Use the tips of fingers for knee stress points. *(Beck, p. 528)*

44.

B. The nervous and endocrine systems are responsible for most stress patterns that can be relieved by disrupting the signals of the sensory receptors. *(Fritz, p. 122)*

45.

A. In Bell's palsy, the paralyzed side of the mouth area is stretched, and massage should be on both sides from the mandible to the hairline in a kneading stroke. *(Beck, p. 195; Tappan, p. 106)*

46.

B. Deep transverse friction should be used to break up scar tissue from overuse in tenosynovitis. *(Tappan, p. 264)*

47.

A. The muscle tissue degenerates during muscular dystrophy as a result of muscle atrophy. *(Beck, p. 123)*

48.

D. Many diseases cause inflammation of tissue and massage is beneficial. They include lupus, spondylitis, and arthritis. *(Fritz, pp. 398–399)*

49.

A. If the level of WBCs becomes lower than normal, the result is leukopenia. *(Tortora, p. 577)*

50.

D. Back pain and tight hamstrings are the result of limited hip and lumbar movement. *(Kapit, p. 54)*

51.

A. The volar area of the wrist is affected in carpal tunnel syndrome. *(Tortora, p. 312)*

52.

A. Lack of muscle movement due to nerve damage is called flaccidity. *(Beck, p. 199)*

53.

A. The median nerve in the arm is responsible for motion and sensation of the thumb, index, and middle finger. If it is cut, the thumb does not have the ability to flex. *(Beck, pp. 199, 209)*

54.

A. Athlete's foot is a fungus infection that attacks the foot and toes. *(Tortora, p. 141)*

55.

D. Rheumatoid arthritis is a chronic inflammatory disease of the joint with cartilage erosion and eventual immobilization. *(Beck, p. 101)*

56.

D. The ulnar nerve travels through the arms, wrists, and fingers. Any injury to this area prevents the function of the wrist or outer fingers. *(Beck, p. 209)*

57.

D. Survivors of abuse benefit from the touch of massage because it triggers many feelings and emotions. *(Ashley, pp. 84–85)*

58.

D. Lumbar pain, a dislocated hip, and a herniated disc are all symptomatic of injury to the sciatic nerve. *(Tortora, p. 398)*

59.
B. Inflammation of the periosteum around the tibia is one symptom of shin splints. *(Tortora, p. 341)*

60.
D. People use chemical substances to help our feelings and in turn alter our emotions, but the use of excess food, drugs, and nicotine can lead to disease. *(Fritz, p. 386)*

61.
C. The receptors of the skin, muscles, and joints can cause somatic pain. *(Fritz, p. 95)*

62.
D. Even though massage is recommended for pregnancy, many contraindications are possible and need a doctor's attention. *(Beck, p. 541)*

63.
D. Any client who suffers from a cardiovascular deviation of any type needs a referral. *(Fritz, p. 404)*

64.
C. Increasing circulation by deep stroking and kneading aids flaccid paralysis in limbs. *(Yates, p. 8)*

65.
D. Myofascial pain includes a plethora of terms: myositis, myofascitis, and fibromyositis. *(Yates, p. 13)*

66.
B. The neurochemicals, endorphins and enkephalins, relieve pain and act as analgesia. *(Yates, p. 25)*

67.
D. Massage therapy is used for whiplash, delivery, neuritis, and neuralgia. *(Yates, p. 27)*

68.
D. A systemic inflammation occurs when an irritant spreads through the body and becomes chronic, such as asthma, arthritis, and bronchitis. *(Fritz, p. 92)*

69.
B. The history intake of an abused client set up mental and physical limits and reassures the client that you will understand. *(Ashley, p. 81)*

70.
D. Pain is difficult to explain or describe because it is a complex of symptoms that include psychological, social, and physiological aspects. *(Fritz, p. 2)*

71.
D. Sunburn has been classified as a first-degree burn. *(Tortora, p. 139)*

72.
A. In second-degree burns, the epidermis and possibly the dermis are damaged. *(Tortora, p. 139)*

73.
D. When the radius is fractured on the distal end, it is classified as a Colles' fracture. *(Tortora, p. 156)*

74.
A. Erosion of the articular cartilage resulting in the bones touching is diagnosed as osteoarthritis. *(Beck, p. 101; Tortora, p. 162)*

75.
B. When assessing passive movement, the springy end feel is the most common. The end feel indicates the presence, type, and severity of lesions in the tissue associated with the joint. *(Beck, p. 437)*

76.
A. Damage to the anterior cruciate ligament of the knee is a very common injury in accidents involving the knee joint. *(Tortora, p. 230)*

77.
B. Neurons do not repair at all when the central nervous system is injured or traumatized. *(Beck, p. 40)*

78.
B. Vesicles are blisters with clear fluid that lie just beneath the epidermis. *(Tortora, p. 5)*

79.
B. The spreading of cancer or metastasis occurs through the blood or lymphatic system. *(Beck, p. 258)*

80.
A. Median nerve damage affects thumb movement and the inability to flex the wrist and pronate the arm. *(Tortora, p. 394)*

81.

D. There are many contraindications to massage including bleeding, swelling, burns, skin infections, tumors, and bruises. *(Beck, p. 259)*

82.

D. Anesthetics block pain so that nerve impulses cannot pass the obstructed region by preventing the opening of the sodium channels. *(Tortora, p. 361)*

83.

D. Epilepsy can be characterized by short, recurrent periodic attacks of motor, sensory, or psychological malfunction as well as seizures, which are initiated by abnormal, synchronous electrical discharges from the brain. A person with epilepsy often times will contract skeletal muscles involuntarily. *(Salvo, p. 258)*

84.

D. Headaches generally occur in the occipital and temporal muscle area. Migraines cannot be helped by analgesics but by drugs that can constrict the blood vessels. *(Tortora, p. 440)*

85.

D. The nerves of the brachial plexus control movement of the arm. *(Beck, p. 199)*

86.

D. Tinnitus is described as the ringing or sounds in the ear as a result of high blood pressure or nerve degeneration. *(Tortora, p. 499)*

87.

D. When the RBCs drop below the normal number, the condition is known as anemia. *(Tortora, p. 568)*

88.

D. When there is a heartbeat more than 100 beats per minute, the result is tachycardia. *(Tortora, p. 630)*

89.

A. The blood can artificially be filtered of wastes by a method called hemodialysis. *(Tortora, p. 891)*

90.

A. Treatment with hot or cold application should not be given if a contraindication is present. *(Beck, p. 471)*

91.

C. The pain-spasm-pain cycle is a result of restricted movement caused by trauma, strain, or injury to the bone, muscle, tendon, or joint. The muscle spasm contracts the muscle that becomes ischemic and that in turn stimulates the pain receptors in the muscle. *(Fritz, p. 94)*

92.

D. When the skeletal muscles contract, the body temperature rises. *(Tortora, p. 854)*

93.

D. The acronym HIV stands for human immunodeficiency virus. *(Tortora, p. 712)*

94.

A. Lordosis is a lumbar curvature of the spine due to poor posture, pregnancy, obesity, or rickets. *(Tortora, p. 195)*

95.

A. Only light massage can benefit the ache and mucous secretion associated with the upper respiratory infections. *(Fritz, p. 407)*

96.

A. Asthma is the disorder that results in the narrowing of the airways as spasms of the smooth muscle close partially or completely (bronchoconstrictor). *(Tortora, p. 756)*

97.

D. Shock is an absolute general contraindication to massage. *(Fritz, p. 393)*

98.

D. The muscles, joints, tendons, fascia, and related areas have receptors that are stimulated from deep somatic pain. *(Fritz, p. 95)*

99.

B. Injuries that cause inflammation to an area should not be massaged. *(Beck, p. 4)*

100.

C. Trigger point therapy palpates small areas of hypertonicity in the muscle associated with myofascial pain, and requires gentle stretching at the end. *(Fritz, p. 101)*

101.

A. In difficult range of motion (ROM) by the client, the therapist to move the body part may provide assistance. *(Beck, p. 325)*

102.

D. When the muscle goes into spasm and cramping results, ice, compression, and cross-fiber friction to contracted muscle provide considerable relief, as well as stretching the spasmed muscle. *(Beck, p. 529)*

103.

A. Any pathogen or open wound on the skin of the client is a contraindication to a massage. There are many contagious skin disorders that can easily be transmitted to the practitioner. A referral to a dermatologist is appropriate. *(Werner & Benjamin, p. 4)*

104.

D. Psoriasis is a chronic skin disease found on the elbows, knees, and trunk. It is non-contagious with accelerated psoriatic skin cell division, which appears pink and scaly. It is only locally contraindicated to acute stages of the disease. *(Werner & Benjamin, p. 26)*

105.

D. Any open wound, sore, or incision as well as any skin disorder related to diabetes is contraindicated. The rule that governs the skin is if the intactness of the skin has been compromised in anyway; the client is susceptible to infection. *(Werner & Benjamin, p. 38)*

106.

A. Gout is a type of arthritis that causes inflammation around the joints of the hands and feet. A diet high in purines is the cause of uric acid crystals forming deposits that result in pain. The kidney is the primary organ that becomes overworked and dysfunctional. *(Werner & Benjamin, p. 75)*

107.

B. The first trimester is when fetal attachment is most fragile and massage therapists must avoid deep abdominal work to prevent any danger to the unborn. *(Werner & Benjamin, p. 349)*

108.

B. Recent studies have shown that breast massage is beneficial to the client, promoting recovery, healing, and range of motion. *(Werner & Benjamin, p. 333)*

109.

D. All hepatitis is contraindicated and should require a note from the physician if it is a chronic case and the liver is stable. *(Werner & Benjamin, pp. 297–299)*

110.

C. Diverticulitis is a protrusion from the wall of the colon that can become infected. Massage is contraindicated. *(Werner & Benjamin, p. 285)*

111.

D. As long as the disease of the common cold, pneumonia, and influenza are in the subacute stage and not the acute stage, massage is not contraindicated. *(Werner & Benjamin, pp. 250–255)*

112.

A. Massage is indicated for *all* stages of HIV clients as long as the practitioner is healthy. *(Werner & Benjamin, p. 234)*

113.

D. Pathogens are transmitted by mucous membrane, broken skin, ingestion, inhalation, and intact skin contaminated with poison ivy, fungus, or scabies. *(Salvo, p. 354)*

114.

D. A massage therapist should wear gloves if the client has broken skin, body fluid, blood lesions, herpes, or requires oral massage. *(Salvo, p. 355)*

115.

D. Scoliosis, contact lenses, and arthritis are not a massage contraindication. Massage is beneficial to any curvature of the spine as well as arthritis. However, it is important to know if a client is wearing contact lenses so that pressure around or on the eye is avoided. *(Salvo, p. 454)*

116.

D. The critical risk factors of breast cancer include, age, genetic predisposition, the female sex, hormonal factors, presence of other cancer, and race.

Although, diet and exercise are important to good health they do not contribute a high risk to cancer. *(Damjanov, p. 396)*

117.

D. Palpatory assessment is through touching with purpose and intent. It is a skill that determines muscle location, temperature of the body, and parts of the body for circulation, fever, inflammation, and restriction in the tissue. *(Salvo, p. 465)*

118.

D. By examining the gait of a client, posture, pain, coordination, and muscle weakness can all be assessed and compared to a normal walking pattern. *(Salvo, p. 468)*

119.

C. Hypoglycemia is a condition when there is not enough glucose in the blood. Massage is indicated, but if the client gets light headed, then assist them off the table and have them eat or drink something. *(Salvo, p. 273)*

120.

C. Anyone with diabetes mellitus can get a massage providing they have taken their medication and the massage is gentle. *(Salvo, p. 273)*

121.

B. The accessory muscles of respiration will be especially tight so focusing on the sternocleidomastoid, scalenes, and pectoralis minor will benefit the client. *(Salvo, p. 312)*

3 Massage Therapy and Bodywork Theory, Assessment, and Practice

OBJECTIVES: Major areas of knowledge/content included in this chapter are based on the NCTMB exam topics and percentage of questions (41%)

1. Assessment

   - Integration of structure and function
   - Use of palpation for assessment of craniosacral pulses, energy blockages, and bony landmarks
   - Using visual cues in assessing client
   - Conventional medical approaches to client's illness
   - Structural compensatory patterns
   - Interview techniques

2. Application

   - Anatomy sites to avoid on client
   - Client draping and supports
   - Physiological and emotional effects of touch
   - Appropriate response to client's needs
   - Universal precautions
   - Appropriate communication skills
   - Physiological changes to touch therapy
   - Self-awareness
   - Use of joint mobilization techniques
   - Use of manual contact and manipulation to affect soft tissue, joints, and the energy system
   - Principles of posture and kinesthetic awareness
   - Hydrotherapy
   - CPR and first aid

1. The most critical skill for developing an optimal client relationship is
   A. Acceptance
   B. Feelings
   C. Listening
   D. Humoring

2. When the client reveals sensitive information and honest thoughts and feelings, this is known as
   A. Self-disclosure
   B. Empathy
   C. Consoling
   D. Moralizing

3. The sequences and directions of Swedish massage strokes are most adapted to which anatomical or physiological situation?
   A. Muscle attachments
   B. Subcutaneous adipose tissue
   C. Autonomic nervous system
   D. Lymph drainage and venous return

4. Which **BEST** describes the effects of massage therapy?
   A. Increased venous and lymph flow
   B. Increased venous, decreased arterial flow
   C. Decreased venous and lymph flow
   D. Decreased venous, increased lymph flow

5. Some road blocks to communication between therapist and client include
   A. Advising and giving solutions
   B. Judging, criticizing
   C. Interpreting, analyzing
   D. All of the above

6. Universal precautions are required when performing
   A. Handling body fluids
   B. Invasive medical procedures
   C. All massage therapy
   D. All of the above

7. When massaging the thigh in the supine position, which is (are) involved?
   A. Hamstrings
   B. Quadriceps
   C. Gluteals
   D. Gastrocnemius

8. The universal precautions were designed by OSHA primarily for the
   A. Clinical massage therapists
   B. Practitioners who handle body fluids
   C. Healthcare workers
   D. All of the above

9. In first aid for a choking victim, you want the conscious victim to
   A. Cough
   B. Swallow
   C. Vomit
   D. Inhale

10. In order to control the spread of pathogenic microorganisms, the therapist should
    A. Wash hands often
    B. Disinfect equipment
    C. Do not massage when ill
    D. All of the above

11. Lymph massage procedures begin at the
    A. Tendons
    B. Left thoracic lymph duct
    C. Right thoracic lymph duct
    D. Immune system

12. Endangerment sites should be avoided during a massage because
    A. They are bilaterally symmetrical
    B. They are areas that can be easily injured
    C. They are areas that are dysfunctional
    D. They are hard to remember

13. A pregnant client should have pillows under her back and knees when she is lying
    A. On her side

B. Supine

C. Prone

D. A and B

14. A pre-event sports massage is shorter with the movements performed

A. Precisely

B. Using heat

C. Slower

D. Faster

15. Cross-fiber massage must be applied in which direction to the fibers?

A. Horizontal

B. Perpendicular

C. Triangular

D. Trapezoidal

16. All the following are endangerment sites **EXCEPT**

A. Popliteal artery

B. Kidney region

C. Brachial plexus

D. Transverse colon

17. In the supine position a bolster is placed under the _____ to take pressure off the lower back.

A. Neck

B. Ankles

C. Knees

D. Sacrum

18. Cold applied for therapeutic purposes is called

A. Cryptology

B. Cryotherapy

C. Ignorance

D. Cool ice

19. The draping method that covers the entire body is called

A. Top-cover

B. Full-sheet

C. Diaper

D. Wrapping

20. In the prone position, support is put under the _____ to ease the pressure on the lower back.

A. Ankles

B. Abdomen

C. Shoulders

D. Chest

21. The draping method that covers the table and wraps the client is called

A. Top-cover

B. Full-sheet

C. Diaper

D. Wrapping

22. Most current massage styles are based on

A. Swedish movements

B. Swiss movements

C. German movements

D. Greek movements

23. Nerve trunks and centers are sometimes chosen as sites for the application of

A. Rolling

B. Rocking

C. Pressure

D. Vibration

24. Support for the cervical area can be provided by a _____ in the supine position.

A. Triangle

B. Face cradle

C. Shoulder cushion

D. Neck roll

25. A bath with a temperature of 85° F to 95° F is considered

A. Cool

B. Cold

C. Tepid

D. Hot

26. The procedure that uses a bouncing movement to improve the flow of lymph through the entire system is called lymphatic
    A. Bounce
    B. Sway
    C. Purging
    D. Pump manipulation

27. The attempt to bring the structure of the body into alignment around a central axis is called
    A. Structural integration
    B. Trauma
    C. Alignment
    D. Adjustment

28. The placement of bolsters in the side lying position are
    A. Head supported with pillow
    B. Under top leg
    C. Under top arm
    D. All of the above

29. When you become a massage therapist you must prepare your _____ and _____.
    A. Balance and flexibility
    B. Strength and stamina
    C. Mind and body
    D. All of the above

30. Realignment of muscular and connective tissue and reshaping the body's physical posture is called
    A. Adjustment
    B. Centering
    C. Rolfing
    D. Posturing

31. A hyperirritable spot that is painful when compressed is called a (an)
    A. Tender point
    B. Pain point
    C. Ampule
    D. Rolfing

32. Self-awareness and self-care for a massage therapist is essential to
    A. Balance our bodies and mind
    B. Offer more to our clients
    C. Maintain balance, strength and stamina
    D. All of the above

33. When you are massaging expose only
    A. The dorsal side
    B. The ventral side
    C. The area being massaged
    D. Sheet being used

34. Better flexibility is the result of
    A. Sustained stretching
    B. Ballistic stretching
    C. Weight lifting
    D. Bicycling

35. Using too much deep pressure causes the muscles to
    A. Have pain
    B. Go limp
    C. Relax
    D. Cramp

36. The general effects of percussion movements are to tone the muscles by
    A. Vibration
    B. Friction
    C. Kneading
    D. Hacking, cupping, slapping, beating

37. A concern with towel draping is it is
    A. Too thick to work with
    B. More difficult to master
    C. Not warm enough
    D. Leaves the abdomen exposed

38. The idea that stimulation of particular body points affects other areas is called
    A. Chiropractic
    B. Reflexology
    C. Rolfing
    D. Touching

39. The stance in which both feet are placed perpendicular to the edge of the table is called the
    A. Archer
    B. Horse
    C. Moose
    D. Stirrup

40. Joint mobilization is a passive movement that can be integrated into a massage routine, for example
    A. Pulling
    B. Friction
    C. Stretching to ROM limit
    D. Tapotement

41. The most difficult part of draping is
    A. Not exposing too much
    B. Covering the body
    C. Turning your client over
    D. Keeping stains off

42. Deep strokes and kneading techniques can cause an increase in
    A. Vasoconstriction
    B. Blood flow
    C. Diastolic arterial pressure
    D. Systolic arterial pressure

43. What **BEST** describes the technique of Rolfing?
    A. Reflex zone therapy
    B. German massage
    C. Structural integration
    D. Neuromuscular massage

44. The cupping technique is best suited for
    A. Acute bronchitis
    B. Cancer of the lungs
    C. Bronchiectasis
    D. Acute tracheitis

45. The method used to turn a client over with sheets is called
    A. Anchor method
    B. Flip method
    C. Turn over method
    D. None of the above

46. An excellent stroke for assessing tissues is
    A. Effleurage
    B. Petrissage
    C. Friction
    D. Tapotement/percussion

47. Beginning anterolaterally on the arm and moving lateral to medial in the anatomical position, the meridians are
    A. ST, LI, TW
    B. LIV, SP, KI
    C. HC, HT, LU
    D. SI, CO, SJ

48. Temperature range for hot immersion baths is **BEST** at
    A. 85° F–95° F
    B. 100° F–110° F
    C. 125° F–150° F
    D. 130° F–140° F

49. Which of the following are used when applying massage strokes?
    A. Intension, pressure, excursion
    B. Rhythm and continuity
    C. Speed, duration, sequence
    D. All of the above

50. The application of force (or thrust) exerted by the massage therapist on the clients body is called
    A. Speed
    B. Depth
    C. Pressure
    D. Excursion

51. In addition to massage, which is most helpful in increasing lymph flow?
    A. Exercise
    B. Heat
    C. Immobilization
    D. Passive movement

52. When applying pressure, it is important to
    A. Not exceed the client's personal pain threshold
    B. Cause muscle relaxation, not contraction
    C. Take into consideration the area on the body where the pressure is applied
    D. All of the above

53. Also referred to as light effleurage, which ancillary stroke is a light finger tracing over the skin to finish a massage therapy?
    A. Pennate
    B. Nerve stroke
    C. Feather friction
    D. Final feathering

54. Localized, sensitive ischemic tissue that is hypersensitive to touch but does not cause referred sensations is
    A. Trigger point
    B. Satellite point
    C. Tender point
    D. Tsubo

55. Stretching that is a combined effort between the therapist and client is known as
    A. Active-passive
    B. Passive-active
    C. Active-assisted
    D. Static-active

56. The therapeutic benefit of friction is
    A. Local hyperemia
    B. Lymphatic drainage
    C. Tonification
    D. None of the above

57. Which meridian is lateral to the midsagittal line of the posterior cervical vertebrae?
    A. Governing vessel
    B. Triple warmer
    C. Stomach
    D. Bladder

58. The main purpose of deep transverse friction is to
    A. Separate muscle fibers
    B. Lengthen muscle fibers
    C. Shorten muscle fibers
    D. Minimize pain

59. A system of active, passive, and resisted movements of the body's various joints and muscles, most often the presentation of passive ROM is called
    A. Active stretching
    B. Table gymnastics
    C. Swedish gymnastics
    D. Passive stretching

60. Which stroke **MOST OFTEN** begins and ends a massage?
    A. Effleurage
    B. Petrissage
    C. Friction
    D. Vibration

61. What is the **BEST** massage technique to lift muscles off the bone?
    A. Effleurage
    B. Petrissage
    C. Vibration
    D. Tapotement

62. Joint movements are traditionally categorized as
    A. Free active and passive
    B. Assistive active and passive
    C. Passive and active
    D. All of the above

63. Stretching that involves the therapist's applying gentle resistance while the client is actively engaging in a stretch is
    A. Active-assisted
    B. Ballistic
    C. Resisted or isometric
    D. Static

64. How should you vary massage treatment time with the age of the patient?
    A. Progressively with increased age
    B. Shorter with increased age
    C. Shorter for very old and very young
    D. The same for any age

65. Which massage technique gives the **BEST** information about connective tissue structure in ligaments, tendons, and joints?
    A. Effleurage
    B. Friction
    C. Vibration
    D. Tapotement

66. Stretching is a type of _____ joint movement that is performed to the limit of the ROM.
    A. Active
    B. Assistive active
    C. Passive
    D. Resistive active

67. Which stroke is **BEST** for breaking down adhesions?
    A. Effleurage
    B. Petrissage
    C. Friction
    D. Vibration

68. In order to challenge the muscles used practitioners apply _____ movement to a joint.
    A. Resistive
    B. Passive
    C. Free
    D. Assistive

69. Strokes that knead are called
    A. Effleurage
    B. Petrissage
    C. Friction
    D. Vibration

70. Joint mobilization techniques are used to help improve
    A. Body alignment
    B. Posture
    C. Reeducating the muscles
    D. All of the above

71. What is the **BEST** stroke for massaging the intercostals?
    A. Compression
    B. Tapotement
    C. Vibration
    D. Petrissage

72. In order to generally assess the degree of flexibility at a joint, the practitioner should have a knowledge of the
    A. Stretch capacity
    B. Normal ROM
    C. Resistive movement
    D. All of the above

73. How should pressure be administered during effleurage?
    A. Evenly
    B. Deep to lighter
    C. Like nerve stroke
    D. Light to deeper

74. Careful joint movement is important in cases of
    A. Metal hardware at the joint
    B. Hip replacement
    C. The elderly
    D. All of the above

75. Biofeedback is useful in
    A. Relieving pain through autogenic training
    B. Controlling involuntary processes
    C. A therapeutic program
    D. All of the above

76. Guided imagery and meditation techniques
    A. Remove blocks and stimulate healing
    B. Are used for preventative treatment
    C. Subliminally reinforce the mind
    D. All of the above

77. Static stretching can be defined as
    A. A stretch performed for 10–15 seconds
    B. Passive movements
    C. A stretch that moves to the point of pain
    D. All of the above

78. Massage can relieve pain without the use of
    A. Imagery
    B. Stimulation
    C. Drugs, alcohol, or narcotics
    D. Endorphins

79. Yoga is a form of mediation for
    A. Good appetite
    B. Muscle balance and relaxation
    C. Dancing
    D. Religion

80. The relaxing action of a muscle is obtained by the application of
    A. Cold
    B. Heat
    C. Neutral
    D. None of the above

81. It is best to stretch a muscle on _____ of the breath.
    A. Exhalation
    B. Holding
    C. Inhalation
    D. Meditation

82. In which massage technique should the fingers move tissue under the skin but not the skin itself?
    A. Tapotement
    B. Effleurage
    C. Vibration

    D. Friction

83. For which type of tissue is vibration the **MOST** unsuitable?
    A. Major nerve course
    B. Reduce muscle spasm
    C. Bony prominences
    D. Skeletal muscle

84. In order to stretch the posterior cervical muscles use the _____ technique with the neck in forward flexion.
    A. Hyperextension
    B. Horizontal flexion
    C. Cross-arm
    D. Finger push-up

85. Which is the first step in beginning massage treatment?
    A. Apply lubricant
    B. Effleurage
    C. Determine contraindications
    D. Diagnose the patient

86. Joint mobilization of the pectoral girdle with the client in the supine position includes all but the following
    A. Shaking
    B. Tapoment
    C. Horizontal flexion
    D. Scissoring

87. First aid for acute soft tissue injuries involves RICE, which means
    A. Ice
    B. Rest and elevation
    C. Compression
    D. All of the above

88. Which aims **MOST** specifically to passively stretch muscle?
    A. Effleurage
    B. Friction
    C. Petrissage

D. Tapotement

89. Massage benefits lymph flow **BEST** when strokes are
   A. Away from heart
   B. Toward heart
   C. Heavy in both directions
   D. In certain local areas

90. For which condition is abdominal massage **MOST** beneficial?
   A. Pregnancy
   B. Appendicitis
   C. Constipation
   D. Enteritis

91. In order to create mobility at the hip joint _____ is used on the leg.
   A. Cupping
   B. Shaking
   C. Rocking
   D. Percussion

92. When the heel of the foot is brought toward the buttocks the _____ muscles are stretched.
   A. Calf
   B. Gluteal
   C. Hamstrings
   D. Quadriceps

93. Which is **BEST** to prevent adhesions in muscle tissue?
   A. Friction and effleurage
   B. Friction and petrissage
   C. Friction and tapotement
   D. Friction only

94. In tapping a large area of the body, which massage maneuver is used?
   A. Percussion
   B. Friction
   C. Effleurage
   D. Petrissage

95. To mobilize the hip through its full ROM bend the leg
   A. Hold for 30 seconds and abduct
   B. Adduct diagonally, extend, abduct diagonally
   C. Circumduct the flexed hip
   D. B and C

96. When applying palmar kneading to calf muscles, with the client in supine position, place a pillow or bolster
   A. Under the sacrum
   B. Under the lower back
   C. Under the knees
   D. Under the ankles

97. Which condition is **ALWAYS** a contraindication for massage?
   A. Muscle spasm
   B. Phlebitis
   C. Rheumatoid arthritis
   D. Edema

98. In order to mobilize the ankle joint under the malleoli of the tibia and fibula
   A. Use a scissoring motion between metatarsals
   B. Dorsiflex the calcaneus
   C. Press the heel of the hands and apply rapid alternate movement of the ankle
   D. Plantar flex the calcaneus

99. In massaging the anconeus, the massage practitioner is working in the area of the
   A. Upper extremity
   B. Lower extremity
   C. Abdominal wall
   D. None of the above

100. For insomnia, which is **BEST**?
   A. Heavy effleurage
   B. Light effleurage
   C. Tapotement
   D. Pick-up

101. A scissoring motion can mobilize the joints of the _____.
    A. Metatarsals
    B. Tarsals
    C. Carpals
    D. Phalanges

102. The main purpose of deep transverse friction is to
    A. Separate muscle fibers
    B. Lengthen muscle
    C. Shorten muscle fibers
    D. Minimize pain

103. Which is characteristic of a pressure stroke?
    A. Is of no consequence
    B. Follows venous flow
    C. Follows arterial flow
    D. Follows force

104. When stretching the intrinsic tissue of the foot
    A. Plantar flex the foot
    B. Interlock fingers between toes
    C. Pull sides of foot away from each other
    D. All of the above

105. A client complains of and requests massage for severe low back pain. Which condition produces this pain and is a contraindication for massage?
    A. Phlebitis
    B. Postural deviation
    C. Herniated disc
    D. Torticollis

106. To massage the hand, use
    A. Effleurage and petrissage
    B. Compression
    C. ROM and circular friction
    D. All of the above

107. The areas of the body for which passive joint movements are effective are
    A. Neck and shoulder girdle
    B. Wrists and hands
    C. Knees, ankles and feet
    D. All of the above

108. To massage the elderly, which stroke would you use?
    A. Tapotement
    B. Gentle effleurage and petrissage
    C. Deep pressure
    D. Friction over pressure area

109. Practitioners use joint movements primarily to
    A. Stimulate production of synovial fluid
    B. Induce muscle relaxation and kinesthetic awareness
    C. Increase joint ROM and muscle strength
    D. All of the above

110. It is essential that the practitioner be knowledgeable about the personal interaction and psychosocial implications of _____.
    A. Structural integration
    B. Touch
    C. Anger
    D. Confidence

111. When palpating the midline of the back, what is being touched?
    A. Transverse process
    B. Vertebral body
    C. Spinal process
    D. Articular joint

112. Mild stimulation of the vagus nerve results in
    A. Irregular heartbeat
    B. No change
    C. Increased heartbeat
    D. Decreased heartbeat

113. Touch by the practitioner is especially important to many special groups of people that include
    A. Victims of sexual abuse
    B. Victims of traumatic stress

C. Victims of physical abuse

D. All of the above

114. Massage therapy is used in pain management for
    A. Cardiac and terminal cancer patients
    B. Post-trauma patients
    C. Post-surgical patients
    D. All of the above

115. The use of cold to depress the activity of pain receptors in the treatment of myofascial pain
    A. Maintains skin temperature of 13.6° C
    B. Increases nerve conduction velocity
    C. Permits passive stretching and exercise
    D. Decreases the general activity of patient

116. Because of the use of touch and the interpersonal nature of massage, the gender issue (s) to be aware of is (are)
    A. Cultural background
    B. Religious background
    C. Cross-gender situations
    D. All of the above

117. The primary physiological effect of massage therapy includes all **EXCEPT**
    A. Delivery of oxygen to cells
    B. Clearance of metabolic waste and by-product of tissue damage
    C. Increased blood and lymph circulation
    D. Increased interstitial fluid and hydro-static pressure

118. Vodder's manual lymph drainage (MLD) was developed for the specific purpose of
    A. Promoting lymph flow from tissue
    B. Eliminating the pneumatic cuff
    C. Decreasing urine output
    D. Increasing erythrocyte count

119. When touch occurs in a sexually sensitive area
    A. It is not a problem
    B. Additional permission is needed

C. Have a consent form signed

D. Professional boundaries are violated

120. The analgesic effect of ice massage is to
    A. Block pain impulse conduction
    B. Reroute pain
    C. Decrease ROM
    D. Eliminate pain

121. Correct lymph massage begins at the
    A. Left thoracic duct
    B. Right arm
    C. Groin
    D. Right thoracic duct at the clavicle

122. Sometimes a recipient's body stores suppressed emotions that may be released in a massage session as
    A. Sighing
    B. Sleeping and snoring
    C. Crying
    D. A and C

123. Communication between practitioner and recipient during a session should be kept
    A. To a minimum
    B. Continuous
    C. Silent
    D. At a whisper

124. The confidential information about the receiver can include
    A. Information during a session
    B. Observations made by the practitioner about physical or emotional condition
    C. Health history
    D. All of the above

125. If a session starts with the recipient in the prone position, a commonly used sequence is
    A. Legs, back, buttocks
    B. Back, buttocks, leg
    C. Buttocks, legs, back
    D. None of the above

126. The purpose of a lubricant when massaging is to
    A. Keep the body greasy
    B. Prevent blisters from forming
    C. Cleanse the body for relaxation
    D. Avoid uncomfortable friction between the therapist's hand and the patient's skin

127. One of the primary purposes of effleurage in massage is
    A. Relaxation
    B. ROM
    C. Spread lubricant
    D. A and C

128. A light compressive force applied to the skin with one hand to release a dysfunction in the connective tissue is associated with
    A. Myofascial releases
    B. craniosacral
    C. Amma
    D. MET

129. If the session starts with the recipient in the supine position, a commonly used sequence is
    A. Head, neck, shoulders and arms, chest, legs, feet
    B. Head, legs, feet, shoulders and arms
    C. Feet, legs, head, chest and arms
    D. Head, arms, chest, legs and feet

130. Neck mobilization in a lateral flexion helps to stretch the cervical muscles and the
    A. Trapezius
    B. Deltoid
    C. Occipital
    D. Rhomboids

131. The all-purpose clean up of bodily fluids is
    A. 2% bleach solution
    B. 10% bleach solution
    C. Distilled water
    D. Concentrated bleach

132. After the massage is complete, the therapist will
    A. Escort the client to the bathroom
    B. Withdraw from the client by using body language
    C. Help dress the client
    D. Ask the client if he did a good job

133. If the session starts with the recipient in the supine position, then after turning the recipient over the generally accepted sequence is
    A. Back, buttock, legs
    B. Legs, buttock, end on back and neck
    C. Back, legs, buttock
    D. None of the above

134. A thorough preliminary client assessment includes
    A. Client history
    B. Client observation
    C. Client examination
    D. All of the above

135. The Trager method uses movement exercises called
    A. Gymnastics
    B. Mentastics
    C. Spirals
    D. Athletics

136. The advantage of starting in the prone position is it
    A. Is warmer
    B. Feels safer to the recipient
    C. Is more comfortable
    D. Is more modest

137. Practitioners use joint movements for a variety of reasons including
    A. To stretch surrounding tissue
    B. To increase range of motion
    C. To increase kinesthetic awareness
    D. All of the above

138. Perform _____ pressure when effleuraging along the tensor fascia latae.
    A. Light
    B. Moderate
    C. Very deep
    D. All of the above

139. When you are turning a recipient and anchoring the sheet
    A. Have the recipient turn away
    B. "Tenting" is commonly done
    C. Avoid tangling
    D. All of the above

140. The various anatomical landmarks for which caution is recommended are _____.
    A. Fragile structures that lie near the surface of the skin
    B. Superficial nerves and blood vessels
    C. Endangerment sites
    D. All of the above

141. A reflex response to massage is that the
    A. Body and nerves respond to stimuli of the sympathetic nervous system
    B. Blood vessels dilate
    C. Blood pressure reduces
    D. All of the above

142. Attentive nurturing touch can be a significant therapeutic factor in treating aging or ill because of its _____ benefits.
    A. Psychosocial
    B. Physical
    C. Mental and emotional
    D. All of the above

143. After cancer surgery, patients may benefit from massage for _____.
    A. Promoting healthy scar tissue
    B. Relieving pain and insomnia
    C. Stress reduction and relaxation
    D. All of the above

144. Connective tissue massage (CTM) is a useful technique for
    A. Preparing for surgery
    B. Psychoemotional status
    C. Loosening tissue following surgery or trauma
    D. Controlling pain

145. Massage is indicated for all but the following
    A. Headaches
    B. Swelling due to lymphedema
    C. Fever
    D. Conditions of nerve entrapment

146. The endangerment sites located at the lateral and medial epicondyle of the humerus include the _____ nerves.
    A. Tibial and radial
    B. Radial and median
    C. Axillary and musculocutaneous
    D. Ulnar and radial

147. Skeletal muscle is affected by massage for which of the following symptoms?
    A. Increased muscle tension
    B. Muscle injury
    C. Spasm or cramp
    D. All of the above

148. What is the term used to describe an observable reddening of the skin resulting from increased blood flow?
    A. Anemia
    B. Hypoxia
    C. Hyperemia
    D. Ischemia

149. The reflex effects of massage are the stimulation of
    A. Motor neurons
    B. Sensory receptors of skin and subcutaneous tissues
    C. Synovial fluid at each joint
    D. Chemotransmitter

150. Ice massage is effective for local pain and
    A. Swelling
    B. Relaxed muscles
    C. Fever
    D. Systemic pain

151. A decrease in blood supply to an organ or tissue is referred to as _____.
    A. Hyperemia
    B. Hypoxia
    C. Anemia
    D. Ischemia

152. Nutrition is an important component to the therapist's wellness training because
    A. Food dictates a work schedule
    B. Without sugar, therapy is not possible
    C. Diet affects the behavior and mood changes
    D. Without fat in a diet the therapist can't stay warm

153. Planning single and multiple client sessions
    A. Is not easy to accomplish initially
    B. Depends on the client history and interview
    C. Depends on the emotional status of the client
    D. Can only be effective after six visits

154. Massage is an indication to the integument or skin layer
    A. Stimulating sebaceous glands
    B. Bringing nutrients to the area
    C. Reducing scar tissue
    D. All of the above

155. The adhesions of a well-healed scar can be broken down between skin tissue by applying
    A. Vibration
    B. Petrissage
    C. Friction
    D. Effleurage

156. To help tone weak muscles by increasing muscle spindle activity _____ is indicated.
    A. Percussion
    B. Effleurage
    C. Tapotement
    D. Friction

157. Massage assists the ease of emotional expression through _____.
    A. Love
    B. Stimulation
    C. Relaxation
    D. Fatiguing the nervous system

158. Reflexology of the hands and feet is based on
    A. Polarity
    B. Trager
    C. Zone therapy
    D. Hydrotherapy

159. A first-aid procedure designed to clear the air passageways of obstructing objects is known as the
    A. Pneumonectomy
    B. Cheyne-Stokes
    C. Cardiopulmonary resuscitation
    D. Heimlich maneuver

160. Massage benefits the nervous system by
    A. Improving skin tone
    B. Eliminating waste material
    C. Relieving pain
    D. Stimulating muscles

161. The application of water (in any form) to the body for therapeutic purposes is called
    A. Floating
    B. Hydrotherapy
    C. Therapy
    D. Washing

162. Massage is indicated for conditions of nerve entrapment that occur when soft tissue constricts the nerve, such as
    A. Carpal tunnel syndrome
    B. Sciatica
    C. Thoracic outlet syndrome
    D. All of the above

163. To ensure a safe and comfortable massage, consider the following
    A. Partial or relative contraindications
    B. Endangerment sites
    C. Absolute contraindications
    D. All of the above

164. During the interview and health history the therapist may discover a pain area and find a need to evaluate the _____ before the massage, to enhance therapeutic goals of the client.
    A. Gait
    B. Posture
    C. SOAP
    D. A and B

165. A mildly stimulating effect is produced by
    A. Standard massage oils
    B. Effervescent tablets
    C. Salt rub
    D. Lavender bath salts

166. Prolonged use of cold applications has which effect?
    A. Stimulating
    B. Energizing
    C. Depressing
    D. Heating

167. Expansion of blood vessels following cold application is called a (an)
    A. Primary effect
    B. Secondary effect
    C. Afterthought
    D. Energizer

168. A full-body steam bath for the purpose of causing perspiration is called a
    A. Swedish bath
    B. Japanese spa
    C. Greek soak
    D. Russian bath

169. A palpatory assessment is essential for documentation of tissue for the following
    A. Feel difference between muscles
    B. Locate origin and insertion of muscle
    C. Assess muscle flexibility, tightness, and tone
    D. All of the above

170. An informed consent contains information from which the clients
    A. Can make decisions for their own protection
    B. Can state the right to cancel treatment
    C. Is advised of benefits/undesirable effects
    D. All of the above

171. Prolonged application of cold leads to a physical condition called
    A. Iglooism
    B. Hyperthermia
    C. Hypothermia
    D. Freezer burn

172. A type of dry heat is a (an)
    A. Ice cube
    B. Microwave
    C. Sauna
    D. Fog

173. Inform the client that a therapist does not _____ medical conditions.
    A. Discipline
    B. Assess
    C. Diagnose
    D. None of the above

174. To integrate the structure and function of the client a _____ assessment helps to evaluate balance and alignment.
    A. Mental
    B. Postural
    C. Ergonomic
    D. B and C

175. Abnormalities in gait are found throughout the postural chain of assessing the following body landmarks
    A. Top of the iliac crests
    B. Top of the fibular heads
    C. Rami of mandible and ears
    D. All of the above

176. Spray showers are effective means of
    A. Calming nerves
    B. Hydrotherapy
    C. Moist heat and mild compression
    D. All of the above

177. Universal precautions are used when administering first aid because
    A. You have to assume that anyone receiving first aid potentially has infectious diseases
    B. HIV is transmitted by exposure to blood and other body fluids
    C. Hepatitis and other pathogens are transmitted by exposure to blood and other body fluids
    D. All of the above

178. Application of cold should be of short duration to prevent tissue injury from
    A. Pain
    B. Thawing
    C. Freezing
    D. Heat

179. To increase circulation to an injured area and promote healing, a therapist can alternate applications of

A. Vibration and friction
B. Feathering and kneading
C. Heat and cold
D. Percussion and feathering

180. The immediate first-aid actions required in treating an injured person are
    A. Talk to the individual, determine if he or she is responsive
    B. If possible, position the individual on the back (unless vomiting)
    C. Call 911 or other EMS, giving the exact location with identifying landmarks, your phone number, nature of the injury, the condition of victim, what is being done, and any other circumstances
    D. All of the above

181. Instead of using a commercial ice pack, put ice cubes into a
    A. Wash cloth
    B. Dish towel
    C. Plastic bag
    D. Bath tub

182. Abnormalities in gait are found through assessing the walking pattern of a client to observe
    A. Placement of the feet
    B. Movement of the hands
    C. Movement of the hips and knees
    D. All of the above

183. When administering first aid, your goal is to obtain all the necessary information related to the injury. You should conduct a primary survey of the situation, which includes
    A. Checking the ABCs (airway, breathing, circulation) and hemorrhaging
    B. Using universal precautions when administering any first aid
    C. Assessing the victim's immediate condition and any unforeseen problems
    D. All of the above

184. Itching, inflammation, sensitivity, or a stinging sensation is considered
    A. Normal
    B. Reasonable
    C. Allergic reactions
    D. Safe

185. A massage table should be stable, firm, and
    A. Tall
    B. Short
    C. Wide
    D. Comfortable

186. The height of a massage table is determined by the
    A. Height of the client
    B. Weight of the client
    C. Practitioner's arm length with palms of hand flat on table
    D. All of the above

187. Avoid using which type of oil in massage?
    A. Sunflower
    B. Mineral
    C. Olive
    D. Apricot

188. In rescue breathing, which of the following is done?
    A. Tilt the head back and lift chin
    B. Pinch nose shut
    C. Seal lips around mouth with two full breaths
    D. All of the above

189. An appropriate hypoallergenic oil combination is
    A. Sesame and almond
    B. Sunflower and canola
    C. Apricot and olive
    D. Peanut and walnut

190. Considerations for designing home therapy for clients with demonstration and return demonstration by the client includes all of the following except
    A. Simple use of only those beneficial and necessary
    B. Fit the clients time, energy and means
    C. Challenge the client
    D. Provide immediate noticeable results

191. Body areas where caution should be used to avoid damaging underlying anatomical structures are called
    A. Contraindications
    B. Endangerment sites
    C. Off limits
    D. Inferior

192. In adult CPR, the pulse is
    A. Not checked
    B. Checked at the wrist
    C. Checked at side of neck
    D. Checked behind knee

193. If a person is suffering from heat cramps,
    A. Do not give liquid with caffeine or alcohol
    B. Do not give any medication
    C. Cool with compresses at neck, groin, and armpits
    D. All of the above

194. The ideal Fahrenheit temperature for a massage room is
    A. 75°
    B. 60°
    C. 90°
    D. 85°

195. Avoid lighting that shines
    A. On the client's legs
    B. On the client's back
    C. On the client's hands
    D. Into the client's eyes

196. When working close to an affected area the circulation is stimulated and promotes
   A. Healing
   B. Blood pressure
   C. Blood sugar
   D. Respiration

197. The first-aid treatment for a seizure is aimed at
   A. Actively restoring consciousness
   B. Protecting victim from injury as it occurs
   C. Calming through massage
   D. Calling for help

198. Direct physical effects of massage techniques on the tissues they contact are called
   A. Reflex effects
   B. Pressure points
   C. Physiological effects
   D. Mechanical effects

199. Which of the following is a local effect of cold therapy?
   A. Vasodilation
   B. Increased circulation
   C. Vasoconstriction
   D. Increased local metabolism

200. The first sign of a person choking is
   A. Pupils dilated
   B. Shallow breathing
   C. Victim cannot answer
   D. Coughing

201. To administer CPR, the victim must
   A. Not be breathing or have a pulse
   B. Be awake
   C. Be able to talk
   D. Be standing

202. The most beneficial use of alternate hot/cold (contrast) treatments is with
   A. Acute muscle spasm
   B. Chronic muscle spasm
   C. Insulin-dependent diabetes
   D. Acute fibromyalgia

203. Alternative methods of stress reduction and relaxation techniques include
   A. Breathing techniques
   B. Visualization
   C. Biofeedback
   D. All of the above

204. In CPR performance, always
   A. Pinch off the nostrils
   B. Keep the head tilted
   C. Watch for the victim's chest to rise
   D. All of the above

205. The therapist may refuse to massage in part or in total a client based upon
   A. The physical appearance or behavior of the client
   B. Information gleaned through the health history and interview process
   C. Inappropriate language or behavior of a sexual nature
   D. All of the above

206. With an unconscious victim, always
   A. Get a chair
   B. Leave in any position
   C. Turn victim on back if lying on a hard surface
   D. Put pillow under head

207. A method to aid stress-related activities is
   A. Wet compresses
   B. Aerobics
   C. Sleep
   D. Deep breathing exercises

208. Massage can enhance
   A. Muscular control
   B. Breathing

C. Relaxation

D. All of the above

209. Meditation is a useful treatment for
    A. Stimulating the flow of natural healing forces
    B. Preventative treatment
    C. Subliminal messages
    D. All of the above

210. The universal distress signal of choking is
    A. Pointing to neck
    B. Rotating neck
    C. Clutching the neck between thumb and index finger
    D. Nodding the head

211. The points to check while practicing massage are
    A. Good body positioning and height
    B. Comfort and relaxation of the patient
    C. Even pressure throughout each stroke
    D. All of the above

212. Variations of effleurage include
    A. Knuckling and stroking
    B. Backstroke and friction
    C. Pressure and brushing
    D. Wide angling and stroking

213. Variations of petrissage include
    A. One-handed petrissage
    B. Open and closed "C" position
    C. "V" hand position
    D. All of the above

214. In the application of the universal precautions issued by the CDC in 1991, massage therapists should avoid contact with
    A. Blood
    B. Vomit
    C. Urine and feces
    D. All of the above

215. The muscle or group that is not included in a massage of the back is
    A. Trapezius
    B. Rhomboids
    C. Pectoralis
    D. Erector spinae

216. During a massage of the abdomen, the patient should
    A. Have hip flexors and abdominal muscles relaxed
    B. Be on his or her side to relax
    C. Be draped completely
    D. None of the above

217. In massaging the upper extremity
    A. Care should be taken at the joints
    B. Popping of joints should be avoided
    C. Stroke from distal to proximal along the brachioradialis
    D. All of the above

218. Massage to the popliteal area requires
    A. Firm deep friction
    B. Gentle working of the gastrocnemius tendon heads
    C. Complete avoidance of space
    D. Petrissage only

219. The *Bindegewebsmassage* is a variation of massage technique that is based on
    A. Massaging the connective tissue under the skin
    B. Cross-fiber friction
    C. Polarity
    D. None of the above

220. In massage, it is important to
    A. Break touch with the client
    B. Apply oil over the entire body
    C. Maintain contact with the client throughout
    D. Prepare the client in a prone position

REVIEW QUESTIONS

221. In massaging the body, it is important to
    A. Drape all parts of the body
    B. Expose only the part to be massaged
    C. Cover the entire body with a sheet
    D. Stand still while delivering technique

222. The Heimlich maneuver is performed by
    A. Pressing the fist into the abdomen with inward thrust
    B. Subdiaphragmatic thrusts
    C. Standing behind victim with arms around waist
    D. All of the above

ANSWERS AND RATIONALES

1.
C. Effective listening means that you understand the emotional state of the sender and that you are focusing attention on receiving the message. *(Salvo, p. 448)*

2.
A. Disclosure of private, sensitive client information without rebuttal and/or judgmental response of the therapist is called self-disclosure. *(Salvo, p. 449)*

3.
D. The principle of Swedish massage is always to massage toward the heart in order to move venous blood and lymph back to the thoracic duct and right atrium. *(Beck, p. 250)*

4.
A. All circulation is improved by massage of muscles stimulating blood back to the heart and circulating lymph through elimination organs. *(Beck, p. 247)*

5.
D. Roadblocks to communication that can cause problems are many, including questioning, analyzing, advising, giving solutions, or interpreting. *(Salvo, p. 449)*

6.
D. Precautions to protect the client and therapist include protective eyewear, vinyl gloves, disinfectants when handling any body fluids or performing an invasive medical procedure. *(Salvo, p. 355)*

7.
B. The quadriceps are the muscles of the anterior thigh in the supine position. *(Beck, p. 409)*

8.
D. OSHA supported and helped to pass federal legislation that requires all healthcare workers who may be exposed to body fluids/waste the protection of universal precautions. *(Salvo, p. 355)*

9.
A. It is best for the choking victim to cough first to attempt removal of obstruction. *(American Red Cross, p. 198)*

10.
D. Transmission of pathogens can be controlled by having good hygiene with clothing, linens and washing hands, disinfecting, and wearing vinyl gloves when necessary. *(Salvo, p. 354)*

11.
C. Lymph massage starts at the right side of the body to drain into the right thoracic lymph duct. Both sides should not be done at the same time. *(Beck, p. 545)*

12.
B. Endangerment sites contain certain anatomical structures that are prone to injury to the client (i.e. blood vessels, nerves, and organs). *(Salvo, p. 440)*

13.
D. Pillows under the back and knees as she lies on her side or supine are more comfortable for a pregnant woman. *(Beck, p. 539)*

14.
D. A pre-event sports massage is a faster, shorter, and more intense technique to prepare the athlete's body for better performance. *(Beck, pp. 515–523)*

15.
B. For cross-fiber massage to be effective on the muscle fibers, application must be perpendicular to spread them apart. *(Tappan, p. 84)*

16.
D. Many nerves, blood vessels, and organ areas are endangerment sites except the colon area is safe to massage for constipation problems. *(Salvo, p. 441)*

17.
C. To minimize the pressure under the lower back place a bolster under the knees. *(Tappan & Benjamin, p. 66)*

18.
B. Cryotherapy is a cold therapy to eliminate pain and allow for massage treatment. *(Beck, p. 464)*

19.
A. A top-cover allows the client to be fully covered by a sheet as well as using a sheet to cover the table. *(Beck, p. 356)*

20.

A. Placing a support under the ankles helps to relieve pressure off the lower back. *(Tappan & Benjamin, p. 66)*

21.

B. The client can be draped using the sheet on the table by lifting it up over the body. *(Beck, p. 356)*

22.

A. Swedish massage is classified as using the fundamental manipulation of massage used today. Most treatments combine one or more of these movements. *(Beck, p. 305)*

23.

D. Vibration treatment follows the path of the nerve: gentle, rhythmical, and fine vibration to the nerve trunk. *(Tappan, pp. 91–92)*

24.

D. In order to support and protect the cervical vertebrae, a neck roll is the most functional bolster. *(Tappan & Benjamin, p. 66)*

25.

C. A tepid (slightly warm) bath is soothing and relaxing, good for nervous and excited people. *(Beck, p. 473)*

26.

D. The lymphatic pump manipulation enhances the flow of lymph and can be done with the lymph drainage massage. Pressure and pumping on the chest is done, 150 bounces per minute, to expel the breath. *(Beck, p. 547)*

27.

A. Structural integration is done by manipulating the fascia of the structural muscles resulting from poor posture and binding of connective tissue. *(Beck, p. 548)*

28.

D. In the side-lying position, support should be provided for the superior leg and arm and under the head to keep the client stationary and comfortable. *(Tappan & Benjamin, p. 67)*

29.

D. A massage therapist must prepare themselves through their mind and body first and then work on their strength, stamina, balance, flexibility, and grounding to become better therapists. *(Salvo, p. 69)*

30.

C. Rolfing is a method of structural integration intended to correctly align the spine and body segments by the use of heavy pressure of knuckles, fist, or elbow into the muscle and connective tissue. *(Beck, p. 549)*

31.

A. Palpating muscles effectively locates tender points and trigger points that are associated with soft tissue pain and dysfunction. *(Beck, p. 439)*

32.

D. Massage therapists need to take care of themselves by balancing the mind and body, maintaining strength and stamina in order to provide more to clients. *(Salvo, p. 368)*

33.

C. Only the area to be massaged should be exposed for privacy as well as warmth to the client. Exposure depends on massage therapy legislation, if any. *(Salvo, p. 382)*

34.

A. The mechanical effect of massage is the stretching of superficial tissue, which encourages better flexibility. *(Tappan, p. 24)*

35.

A. Deep pressure techniques such as Rolfing must be done with caution to avoid too much pain. *(Beck, p. 309)*

36.

D. Hacking, cupping, slapping and beating are all forms of quick percussion to tone muscles. *(Beck, p. 311)*

37.

B. It is more difficult to work with a towel due to its size over the body and what it can cover. Practice is required to develop this skill. *(Salvo, p. 382)*

38.
B. Organs and functions of the body can be affected by pressing reflex zones on the hands and feet. The technique is reflexology. *(Tappan, p. 255)*

39.
B. The foot positions in posture and stances aid balance and allow a more direct delivery of massage strokes. The horse is a common one in which both feet are placed perpendicular to the table. *(Beck, p. 336)*

40.
C. Stretching is used to mobilize and increase the flexibility at the joint as it elongates the muscle and connective tissue. *(Tappan, p. 107)*

41.
C. The greatest challenge to a massage therapist is keeping the drape securely in place when turning the client over, since this is when accidental exposure can take place. *(Salvo, p. 383)*

42.
B. Any deep pressure strokes stimulate the circulation and therefore blood flow. *(Beck, p. 253)*

43.
C. Rolfing aligns the major body segments through fascia manipulation to establish structural integration. *(Beck, p. 16)*

44.
C. Congestive lung conditions are treated with the cupping technique of percussion. *(Beck, p. 324)*

45.
A. The anchor method allows for the privacy of the client to turn while the therapist holds the top sheet up to their shoulders and anchors the bottom of the sheet with their thighs against the table. *(Salvo, p. 384)*

46.
A. Effleurage is the first and most frequent used Swedish stroke and its gliding movements are excellent for assessing the client's body and tissue. *(Salvo, p. 400)*

47.
A. The stomach, large intestine, and triple warmer are meridians that travel from the lateral arm to the median part of the anterior body. *(Tappan, pp. 137–139)*

48.
B. The temperature best for nerves, insomnia, and aching muscles is 100° F–110° F. This induces relaxation and relieves nervous tension. *(Beck, p. 473)*

49.
D. The elements involved in applying a skillful massage are a blend of strokes, biomechanics, your intention, pressure, rhythm, speed, duration, and sequence. *(Salvo, p. 397)*

50.
C. Pressure is the application of force exerted by the massage therapist. The pressure should start light and gradually add more until desired effect is achieved. *(Salvo, p. 398)*

51.
A. Exercise stimulates lymph flow due to muscle contracting on the lymph vessels, forcing the movement of the lymph. *(Beck, p. 544)*

52.
D. The sensation of pressure can be very beneficial by the stimulation of compression of the body's surface and cause relaxation. *(Salvo, p. 398)*

53.
B. The light touches over an area that has just been massaged ends with a finger light nerve stroke with clothes on or off. *(Salvo, p. 414)*

54.
C. A tender point is not considered a trigger point because the site causes no referred sensations. *(Salvo, p. 416)*

55.
C. Therapeutic stretching is performed by changing the joint position in order to lengthen the specific muscle. Active-assisted stretching is between the therapist and client actively. *(Salvo, p. 420)*

56.

A. A form of friction called compression increases circulation and lasting hyperemia in the tissue. The pumping action brings blood to deep muscles for long periods. *(Beck, p. 320)*

57.

D. The bladder meridian is lateral to the mid-sagittal line of the posterior cervical vertebrae. *(Beck, p. 566)*

58.

A. To separate muscle fibers from an injury or scar, transverse friction is the recommended therapy. *(Beck, p. 318)*

59.

C. Swedish gymnastics includes the artful and fluid presentation of passive ROM that includes table stretches and joint mobilization. *(Salvo, p. 423)*

60.

A. The stroke that usually begins and ends a massage is effleurage. *(Beck, p. 312)*

61.

B. Petrissage is the best stroke to lift the muscle off the bones. *(Beck, p. 316)*

62.

D. Joint mobilizations are performed within the normal range of joint movement and include active (i.e., free or assistive) and passive movements, which can be integrated into a massage routine. *(Tappan & Benjamin, p. 107)*

63.

C. Even though isometric stretches are not contraction the resistance enhances flexibility and blood flow, which results in relaxation. *(Salvo, p. 422)*

64.

C. Treatment to the old and young should be shortened. They are more fragile and cannot endure a lengthy session. *(Beck, p. 77)*

65.

B. Friction allows the fingers to feel the tissues below due to the deeper pressure applied. *(Beck, p. 319)*

66.

C. Stretching is a type of passive joint movement that can be performed to move a joint to the ROM limit. *(Tappan, p. 107)*

67.

C. To loosen adhesion tissue, cross-fiber friction is the best stroke to mobilize the area. *(Beck, p. 318)*

68.

A. In resistive movement, practitioners offer resistance to the movement thereby challenging the muscles used. *(Tappan, p. 107)*

69.

B. In the petrissage stroke, the tissue is lifted up off the bone in a kneading technique. *(Beck, p. 315)*

70.

D. Body alignment, posture, and reeducating the muscles are all assets of joint mobilization. *(Tappan & Benjamin, p. 108)*

71.

A. Compression is an excellent massage for the intercostal muscles of the ribs. The pumping action provides improvement of breathing. *(Beck, p. 533)*

72.

B. Knowledge of the normal ROM is essential to assess the degree of flexibility at a joint. *(Tappan & Benjamin, p. 108)*

73.

A. The pressure during effleurage should be done evenly from the beginning to the end of the stroke. *(Beck, p. 347)*

74.

D. To ensure safe joint movement, in the cases of elderly and joint replacement or metal inserts, it is important to understand the condition from medical records or the recipients physician. *(Tappan & Benjamin, p. 108)*

75.

D. Biofeedback has many therapeutic uses, including pain relief through autogenic training and aid in controlling involuntary processes. *(Tappan, p. 48)*

76.

D. Imagery and meditation are techniques used to remove blocks, stimulate healing, and subliminally reinforce the mind. *(Tappan, p. 50)*

77.

D. Holding a stretch to a limit to pain is passive movement and a static stretch. *(Tappan & Benjamin, p. 109)*

78.

C. Massage can relieve pain without the use of drugs, alcohol, or narcotics. *(Tappan, p. 45)*

79.

B. When yoga is practiced, the result can be muscle balance and relaxation. *(Beck, p. 603)*

80.

B. Heat to the muscle area stimulates the muscle to relax. *(Beck, p. 460)*

81.

A. Breathing may be used to help the recipient relax during a stretch during the process of exhaling. *(Tappan & Benjamin, p. 109)*

82.

D. Friction is the massage stroke that moves the fascia and tissue under the skin without moving the skin itself. *(Beck, p. 318)*

83.

C. Bony prominences are too sensitive for vibration massage. *(Beck, p. 324)*

84.

C. The cross-arm stretch is the best technique for cervical muscles by lifting the head with one hand and placing other hand across it to the shoulder. *(Tappan & Benjamin, p. 111)*

85.

C. All contraindications should be determined before giving a massage treatment. *(Beck, p. 253)*

86.

D. Scissoring motion is used to create movement between the metacarpals of the joints. *(Tappan & Benjamin, p. 120)*

87.

D. RICE is an acronym for rest, ice, compression, and elevation. *(Beck, p. 522)*

88.

A. Effleurage is the massage stroke that passively moves and stretches muscles. *(Beck, p. 310)*

89.

B. A benefit of massage is that, when the stroke is toward the heart, blood drains from the venous system and lymph from the lymphatic. *(Beck, p. 183)*

90.

C. A benefit of abdominal massage is alleviating constipation. *(Beck, p. 414)*

91.

C. Rocking the leg is a good technique to mobilize the hip joint. *(Tappan & Benjamin, p. 128)*

92.

D. Stretching the quadriceps muscles is accomplished by bringing the foot to the gluteal area. *(Tappan & Benjamin, p. 127)*

93.

A. Friction and effleurage can prevent scarring and adhesions to muscle tissue due to the action of keeping the fiber separated by either cross-fiber or longitudinal strokes. *(Beck, p. 319)*

94.

A. Percussion includes tapping, slapping, hacking, cupping, and beating, which benefit a large area like the back. *(Beck, p. 492)*

95.

D. A full ROM for hip flexion is adduction, extend and abduct the knee diagonally to circumduct the hip completely. *(Tappan & Benjamin, p. 122)*

96.

C. When the client is in the supine position, a pillow or bolster is placed under the knees so that palmar kneading is possible. *(Beck, p. 373)*

97.

B. Phlebitis is always a contraindication for massage. Inflammation in the veins or a possible clot is a dangerous condition. *(Beck, p. 256)*

98.

C. With the recipient supine, the ankle can be mobilized by placing the heel of the hands on the foot under the malleoli and pressing in alternating one side then the other. *(Tappan & Benjamin, p. 128)*

99.

A. Extending the elbow is the action of the anconeus in the upper arm, which originates on the humerus. *(Beck, p. 129)*

100.

B. Light strokes to the forehead are good for nervous headaches and insomnia; gentle gliding strokes are beneficial. *(Beck, p. 312)*

101.

A. To mobilize the tissues between the metatarsals, use the scissoring motion by taking the knuckles of two toes and move up and down. *(Tappan & Benjamin, p. 129)*

102.

A. The transverse action of friction is applied across muscle and tendon to separate fibers, allowing greater circulation and increased mobility. *(Beck, p. 318)*

103.

D. The slightest pressure is transmitted to deeper muscles by force. *(Beck, p. 313)*

104.

D. The intrinsic tissues of the foot can be stretched by interlocking fingers between the toes, pulling the sides of the foot away from each other, and plantar flexing the foot. *(Tappan & Benjamin, p. 130)*

105.

C. When the fibrocartilage of the intervertebral disc is herniated, lower lumbar pain contraindicates massage in that area of the back. *(Tortora, p. 195)*

106.

D. A complete massage to the hand is effleurage, circular friction to the back of the hand, petrissage, ROM, and compression to wrist and fingers. *(Beck, p. 400)*

107.

D. Passive joint movements are effective on most of the body's major joints including neck, shoulder, chest, wrists, hands, hip, knees, ankles, and feet. *(Tappan & Benjamin, p. 131)*

108.

B. Gentle massage is beneficial to the elderly, even if they are frail. *(Beck, p. 259)*

109.

D. Joint mobilization is used and incorporated into a massage routine to relax muscles, stimulate synovial fluids, increase ROM, and kinesthetic awareness. *(Tappan & Benjamin, p. 131)*

110.

B. Touch is the number one skill a practitioner giving a massage needs. To touch is to come in contact with and communicate feelings. *(Tappan & Benjamin, p. 58)*

111.

C. The spinal process runs along the midline of the back when palpating the line of the vertebra. *(Tortora, p. 319)*

112.

D. The vagus nerve is the tenth cranial nerve, which acts as a decelerator of the heartbeat. *(Tortora, p. 611)*

113.

D. Because many men and women have been victims of sexual and physical abuse and traumatic stress, these people need special care regarding touch. The practitioner should make the recipient feel especially safe and comfortable. *(Tappan & Benjamin, p. 58)*

114.

D. Massage therapy is used for post-trauma and post-surgical patients, as well as for cancer and cardiac patients. *(Yates, p. 27)*

115.

C. Cold depresses pain receptors, allowing treatment by passive stretching. *(Yates, p. 27)*

116.
D. The gender issues to be aware of are a person's cultural or religious background as well as the issues of cross-gender massage. *(Tappan & Benjamin, p. 59)*

117.
D. Interstitial fluid and hydrostatic pressure increases are not significant physiological effects of massage. *(Yates, p. 1)*

118.
A. To shift edema fluid from tissues to blood, Vodder (in 1965) designed the MLD (manual lymph drainage). *(Yates, p. 3)*

119.
D. Permission to touch a sexually sensitive area for therapeutic purposes should have the client's consent. *(Tappan & Benjamin, p. 61)*

120.
A. Ice is used to block pain before massaging an area. *(Yates, p. 26)*

121.
D. The right thoracic duct is the correct place to start lymph massage. *(Beck, pp. 544–547)*

122.
D. As a recipient relaxes and lets down emotional defenses they may release a sigh or start crying. This is normal and should not stop a session. *(Tappan & Benjamin, p. 60)*

123.
A. Conversation should be kept to a minimum so that the body and mind can relax. *(Tappan & Benjamin, p. 61)*

124.
D. In a professional relationship there is implicit trust that the practitioner will keep confidentiality about medical and health history as well as observations made about the recipient before, during, or after a session. *(Tappan & Benjamin, p. 61)*

125.
B. The common sequence for the prone position first is the back, buttocks, and legs before the recipient is turned over. *(Tappan & Benjamin, p. 134)*

126.
D. A lubricant avoids an uncomfortable friction on the skin of the patient. *(Tappan, p. 14)*

127.
D. Spreading of the lubricant and muscle relaxation results from the flow of the effleurage stroke. *(Tappan, p. 69)*

128.
A. The movement of connective tissue is known as myofascial therapy used by John Barnes and John Upledger. *(Fritz, p. 367)*

129.
A. The head and neck are started in the supine position. Then the shoulders and arms, chest and abdomen and legs and feet are finished before turning the recipient over. *(Tappan & Benjamin, p. 134)*

130.
A. Only the trapezius is stretched with a lateral flexion of the neck. *(Tappan, p. 111)*

131.
B. A 10% bleach solution is the clean up for HIV, hepatitis, and viral organisms. The solution is one-cup bleach to one gallon of water. *(Fritz, p. 115)*

132.
B. The massage therapist will move away from the client when the massage is complete so that it is understood that the session is over. *(Fritz, p. 35)*

133.
B. When you start a session supine and turn over to the prone position the sequence is generally legs, buttocks, and end with the back and neck. Either way you start, you should end at the head. *(Tappan & Benjamin, p. 134)*

134.
D. Client assessment includes a history, observation, and an examination. *(Beck, p. 295)*

135.
B. Mentastics is the gentle rocking or shaking of body parts, called the Trager method. *(Beck, p. 16; Tappan, p. 299)*

136.

B. It generally feels safer to the recipient to start prone, especially if it is a first time massage. *(Tappan & Benjamin, p. 134)*

137.

D. Movement of the joints stimulates muscle relaxation, increases ROM and kinesthetic awareness, as well as stretching surrounding tissue and stimulating production of synovial fluid. *(Tappan, p. 111)*

138.

B. Moderate pressure can be applied to the IT band and the tensor fascia latae due to its length and strength. *(Tappan & Benjamin, p. 138)*

139.

D. The recipient turns away from the practitioner under a tenting of the sheet which avoids tangling in the sheet. *(Tappan & Benjamin, p. 140)*

140.

D. Endangerment sites include areas of the body that are fragile to the touch and lie superficial to the surface of the skin such as nerves and blood vessels. *(Salvo, p. 430)*

141.

D. The sympathetic nervous system responds as a reflex of the blood vessel dilation, muscle relaxation, and lowering of the resting blood pressure. *(Salvo, p. 430)*

142.

D. There are many benefits to treating the aging or dying through touch. It can improve physical, mental, and emotional functioning as well as ease some of the pain and anxiety felt. *(Tappan & Benjamin, p. 343)*

143.

D. Although massage is generally contraindicated for cancer patients, it has been found the post-surgery massage has many benefits including, stress reduction and relaxation, relieving pain and insomnia, and increasing ROM. *(Tappan & Benjamin, p. 349)*

144.

C. CTM improves circulation and post-operative ANS reflexes that increase sympathetic nerve activity. *(Yates, p. 6)*

145.

C. Fever, or pyrexia is a contraindication for massage therapy because of the risk of spreading infection. *(Salvo, p. 438)*

146.

D. The ulnar and radial nerves of the medial and lateral epicondyles of the humerus are considered nerve endangerment sites because they are superficially located. *(Salvo, p. 442)*

147.

D. The muscle responds to massage after an injury, spasm, or tension. *(Yates, p. 10)*

148.

C. The release of histamines and acetylcholine cause dilation of blood vessels called hyperemia. *(Salvo, p. 431)*

149.

B. Stimulation of the sensory receptors of the skin is the reflex effect of massage. *(Tappan, p. 33)*

150.

A. Swelling can be reduced by ice packs. *(Beck, p. 467)*

151.

D. Muscle pain is a result of a decreased supply of blood to the tissue or an organ called ischemia. *(Salvo, p. 431)*

152.

C. One wellness component is taking care of the body through nutrition to help prevent fatigue and mood changes from cravings. *(Fritz, pp. 382–383)*

153.

B. After a thorough history intake and verbal interview, the therapist can develop a plan of action. *(Fritz, p. 15)*

154.

D. Massage improves the skin color, texture, stimulation of oil secretion, and reduction of adhesions or scar tissue. *(Salvo, p. 432)*

155.

C. Friction of the cross-fibers is an excellent method to break down well-healed scar adhesions. *(Tappan, p. 83)*

156.

C. Tapotement (a form of vibration) creates minute muscle contractions to help tone weak muscles. *(Salvo, p. 433)*

157.

C. A psychological effect of massage is relaxation to ease emotional expression. *(Salvo, p. 436)*

158.

C. Different organs and parts of the body respond to reflex zones in the hands and feet. *(Tappan, p. 255)*

159.

D. The Heimlich maneuver (abdominal thrust) is the first-aid procedure to force air or water out of the trachea or lungs. *(Tortora, p. 761)*

160.

C. Massage techniques have an effect on reflex reaction to relieve pain. *(Beck, p. 249)*

161.

B. Water in the form of ice, liquid, or steam vapor with massage has a therapeutic effect on the body. *(Beck, p. 469)*

162.

D. Conditions of the nervous system that are indicated for massaging areas of nerve entrapment are carpal tunnel and thoracic outlet syndromes and sciatica. *(Salvo, p. 436)*

163.

D. It is essential to heed caution to ensure that the massage is safe and comfortable, therefore partial or relative contraindications, endangerment sites, and absolute contraindications must all be considered. *(Salvo, p. 440)*

164.

D. The therapist should examine and evaluate the gait and posture of a client with pain in order to proceed with caution and knowledge. *(Salvo, p. 464)*

165.

C. Salt rubs are stimulating to the skin and increase some circulation as well. *(Beck, p. 470)*

166.

C. Nerve sensitivity is depressed. *(Beck, p. 472)*

167.

B. Blood vessels constrict initially after cold application. *(Beck, p. 473)*

168.

D. A steam room for cleansing and relaxing provides a Russian bath. *(Beck, p. 481)*

169.

D. A palpatory assessment is important before a massage to document the client's soft tissue. The muscle type, structure, flexibility and tone all add to the style of the massage session. *(Salvo, p. 465)*

170.

D. Information in an informed consent helps the client to have knowledge and decision making rights. *(Salvo, p. 460)*

171.

C. Extreme cold should be of short duration because the tissue temperature lowers. *(Beck, p. 464)*

172.

C. Heat in a sauna room is always produced by a dry heat source of 120° F. *(Beck, p. 463)*

173.

C. A therapist cannot diagnose any medical condition. *(Salvo, p. 460)*

174.

D. A postural or ergonomic assessment studies the anatomy and physiology as it relates to the balance and alignment of the client. *(Salvo, p. 468)*

175.

D. Assess symmetry by placing one finger on a bony landmark and draw an imaginary line bilaterally across the ears, eyes, shoulders, hips, patella, malleoli, and foot arches. *(Salvo, p. 468)*

176.

D. Spray showers have many hydrotherapeutic effects. *(Beck, p. 462)*

177.
D. Potential disease or infection can be transmitted when administering first aid. *(American Red Cross, p. 29)*

178.
C. The tissue freezes if it is too cold too long. *(Beck, p. 464)*

179.
C. Heat and cold are the most effective methods of promoting healing through circulation. *(Beck, p. 469)*

180.
D. Call 911 or EMS. Talk to the person to get a response. *(American Red Cross, p. 29)*

181.
C. A sealable plastic bag makes an excellent ice pack. *(Beck, p. 465)*

182.
D. Observe a "normal" walking pattern and notice the movement of the client's hands, hips, knees, and feet to determine any abnormalities in the gait. *(Salvo, p. 469)*

183.
D. Check ABCs (airway, breathing, and circulation) and hemorrhaging and administer first aid. *(American Red Cross, p. 19)*

184.
C. These signs indicate sensitivity to skin to result in an allergic reaction. *(Beck, p. 277)*

185.
D. A table should be comfortable with padding to absorb pressure applied by practitioners. *(Beck, p. 274)*

186.
C. To prevent fatigue, the palm of a hand should be flat on the table with arms straight. *(Beck, p. 273)*

187.
B. Mineral oils are not recommended because they are petroleum-based, dry the skin, and clog pores. *(Beck, p. 276)*

188.
D. Rescue breathing requires tilting the head, pinching the nose, and breathing into the mouth twice. *(American Red Cross, p. 199)*

189.
B. Mild oils, such as sunflower and canola, are appropriate, hypoallergenic and easy to work with. Oils of nuts can cause allergic reactions. *(Beck, p. 276)*

190.
C. It is not a good plan to design a home plan that will challenge the client, the design should be to get results and build confidence. *(Salvo, p. 471)*

191.
B. Endangerment sites are major nerves, blood vessels, and vital organs that, if exposed to deep pressure, can cause possible injury. *(Beck, p. 265)*

192.
C. In CPR the pulse is checked at the carotid artery at side of neck. *(American Red Cross, p. 203)*

193.
D. For heat cramps, never give coffee, alcohol, or medication. Cool the person down at the neck, groin, and armpits. *(American Red Cross, p. 156)*

194.
A. The temperature of the room must be warm enough for the client and cool enough for the practitioner. *(Beck, p. 272)*

195.
D. Indirect, soft natural light is most desirable, especially for the eyes. *(Beck, p. 272)*

196.
A. By working on areas that have been injured or affected by over exercising, healing, and circulation are improved. *(Beck, pp. 507–508)*

197.
B. Protect the victim from injury during a seizure. *(American Red Cross, p. 169)*

198.

D. The mechanical effects of massage are directly related to the physical strokes and techniques used. *(Beck, p. 506)*

199.

C. The initial effect of cold is vasoconstriction, which chills the skin and contracts the blood vessels to limit swelling. *(Beck, p. 472)*

200.

C. The first sign of a person choking is that he or she cannot answer. *(American Red Cross, p. 199)*

201.

A. CPR can be administered to a victim who is not breathing or does not have a cardiac pulse. *(American Red Cross, p. 205)*

202.

B. For chronic muscle spasms, use alternate hot/cold (contrast) to increase local circulation, relieve chronic pain, and aid healing. *(Beck, p. 469)*

203.

D. Biofeedback, breathing for relaxation, and visualization are all stress reducers. *(Beck, pp. 602–605)*

204.

D. In CPR it is important to pinch off the nostrils, tilt the head back, and observe the victim's chest. *(Teaguarden, p. 37)*

205.

D. Any behavior or language that is inappropriate is a reason for the therapist to refuse massage. *(Salvo, p. 472)*

206.

C. Always turn an unconscious victim on the back before administering CPR, unless victim is vomiting. *(Teaguarden, p. 48)*

207.

D. Deep breathing exercise is a method to aid stress-related activities. *(Beck, p. 602)*

208.

D. Massage enhances muscle control, breathing, and relaxation and can complement a yoga meditation session. *(Beck, p. 603)*

209.

D. Meditation is a treatment for stimulating the flow of natural healing forces, preventative treatment, as well as receiving subliminal messages. *(Tappan, p. 50)*

210.

C. Clutching the neck between the thumb and index finger is the universal distress signal of a choking victim. *(Teaguarden, p. 42)*

211.

D. Good massage techniques include checking patient comfort, even pressure when stroking, and good body positioning. *(Tappan, p. 71)*

212.

A. Knuckling and stroking are variations of effleurage. *(Tappan, p. 73)*

213.

D. The petrissage stroke varies as a "V" hand position, open and closed "C" position, and a one-handed petrissage. *(Tappan, p. 78)*

214.

D. The universal precautions were issued to prevent the spread of bacteria and virus. Therefore, contact with the client's blood, urine, feces, and vomit should be avoided. *(Fritz, p. 113)*

215.

C. The back does not contain the pectoralis muscle, which is the primary chest muscle. *(Tappan, p. 98)*

216.

A. Always relax the hip flexors and abdominal muscles when massaging the abdominal area. *(Tappan, p. 97)*

217.

D. When massaging the upper limbs, care should be taken with the movement of the joints and strokes should go from distal to proximal along the brachioradialis. *(Tappan, pp. 98–100)*

218.

B. The popliteal area of the posterior leg should be gently massaged at the gastrocnemius tendon heads due to the presence of blood vessels and nerves in the area. *(Tappan, p. 102)*

219.

A. The massage that concentrates on the connective tissue under the skin is the *Bindegewebsmassage.* *(Tappan, p. 220)*

220.

C. Strokes should be continuous and maintained without breaks in contact. The client can become startled with reestablishing contact. *(Beck, p. 373)*

221.

B. Expose the area to be massaged, but keep the rest of body draped for privacy and professionalism. *(Beck, p. 372)*

222.

D. The procedure for the Heimlich maneuver is to stand behind the victim and apply subdiaphragmatic thrusts into the abdomen with the fists. *(Teaguarden, p. 42)*

CHAPTER

4 Professional Standards, Ethics, and Business Practices

OBJECTIVES: Major areas of knowledge/content included in this chapter are based on the NCTMB exam topics and percentage of questions (12%)

1. NCTMB Code of Ethics

2. Confidentiality

3. Interprofessional communication

4. Income-reporting procedures

5. Business and accounting practices

6. Session record-keeping practices

7. Scope of practice: legal and ethical parameters

1. The purpose of a client-practitioner agreement is to
   A. Develop clarity as to the nature of service
   B. Protect from unrealistic expectations
   C. Act as a consent reinforcement
   D. All of the above

2. When screening new clients it is important to
   A. Design a questionnaire to ensure you get information desired
   B. Determine if the client has special needs
   C. Determine the expectations of the client
   D. All of the above

3. The letters SOAP refer to
   A. Scale, office, access, plan
   B. Subjective, open, area, parameter
   C. Social, object, active, plan
   D. Subjective, objective, assessment, plan

4. When someone calls requesting sexual services
   A. Hang up and get caller ID
   B. Explain the nature of the profession and the services you provide
   C. Stay centered in your professionalism
   D. B and C

5. Many massage therapists are confronted with obstacles that diminish the drive and motivation of a new business such as
   A. Burnout
   B. Start-up costs
   C. Lack of advertising knowledge
   D. All of the above

6. In business, phone etiquette is important because
   A. It makes an impression of who you are ethically and professionally
   B. It conveys how you feel about your practice
   C. The phone call is taped
   D. A and B

7. If a client's condition is outside the massage technician's scope of practice, the technician should
   A. Schedule extra sessions
   B. Refer the client to the proper professional care
   C. Take more training
   D. Read textbooks to learn more

8. Clear written contracts are an integral part of a business relationship because
   A. They provide a predetermined method to resolve problems
   B. They help avoid problems
   C. They keep you focused on your goals
   D. All of the above

9. If you are planning to be an independent contractor
   A. You are paid in regular intervals (i.e., hour, week, month)
   B. You are reimbursed for travel expenses
   C. You must provide your own table, linens, lotion, etc.
   D. You can be discharged by the employer

10. Reviewing records before a client's visit refreshes your memory and gains the client's
    A. Sympathy
    B. Information
    C. Trust
    D. Dependence

11. If you are planning to be an employee IRS requires that you
    A. Have been trained by the business to perform services
    B. Have no investment in the facility
    C. Can receive expenses and pay at regular intervals
    D. All of the above

12. All client information should be considered above all
    A. Essential

B. Important

C. For the record

D. Confidential

13. Examples of common ethical dilemmas in the health care profession is (are)

A. Inappropriate advertising

B. Breaking confidentiality

C. Practicing beyond your scope

D. All of the above

14. The NCTMB code of ethics is designed to

A. Promote respect for the dignity of persons

B. Promote integrity in relationships

C. Promote responsible caring for clients

D. All of the above

15. A professional code of ethics includes all but the following

A. Post credentials and policies

B. Maintains confidentiality

C. Adhere to city, county and state requirements

D. Charge any price for services

16. When opening a massage business, helpful resources include

A. Chamber of Commerce

B. Accountant

C. Small Business Administration

D. All of the above

17. Pricing a service business such as massage therapy is (are) based on

A. Assets and cash flow

B. Capitalized earnings

C. Net present value and future earnings

D. All of the above

18. If a massage therapist is found guilty of violation of the Massage Practice Act or Rules of Conduct, which action should be taken?

A. Warning only

B. Suspension of license

C. Revocation of license

D. All of the above

19. The major benefit (s) in good interprofessional communication is (are)

A. Client retention

B. Referrals

C. Quality therapeutic results

D. All of the above

20. Business expenses can include the cost of

A. Business cards and advertising

B. Professional clothes and linens

C. License, insurance, and memberships

D. All of the above

21. What is the importance of documenting your work and keeping files

A. You can't count on your memory

B. Keeps you informed of clients needs

C. Record keeping is necessary for IRS

D. All of the above

22. Client files are important for

A. Record keeping for the Internal Revenue Service

B. Keeping well informed of client's needs

C. Documenting your work on clients

D. All of the above

23. Techniques to market professional skills include

A. Publications and presentations

B. Business cards and brochures

C. Donation of services

D. All of the above

24. A typical client intake form should include

A. Name and address

B. Name, address, occupation, physician, emergency number

C. Name, phone, hobbies

D. Name, marital status, children

25. A massage therapist or bodyworker can claim business deductions on Schedule C for
    A. Cost of massage table, linens, and oils
    B. All vacations
    C. Professional convention fees
    D. A and C

26. In opening a massage office, it is essential to investigate certain requirements including
    A. Zoning
    B. Fire inspection
    C. Licensing laws
    D. All of the above

27. SOAP charting is being widely adopted by massage professionals because
    A. Use of a professional reporting system enhances the image of massage as a valuable therapy
    B. Other health care professionals cannot understand the language
    C. It can be used in a court of law
    D. Clients want a record of their health

28. A ledger that separates and classifies every business expenditure is called a (an)
    A. Inventory
    B. Disbursement record
    C. Voucher
    D. Tax ID

29. A good way to save on advertising is to
    A. Make up client referral cards with a discount
    B. Use the yellow pages
    C. Send out flyers
    D. Purchase name lists to solicit

30. Many massage therapists and bodyworkers are
    A. Entrepreneurs
    B. Partners
    C. Sole proprietors
    D. Employers

31. If you choose to work for insurance reimbursement
    A. Thorough documentation is necessary
    B. Your treatment must be medically necessary
    C. You need a letter of referral from the physician
    D. All of the above

32. A record of monies owed to you by others is called
    A. Charges
    B. Accounts receivable
    C. Statements
    D. Liabilities

33. The insurance company(s) that a massage therapist can submit a claim to is (are)
    A. Workers compensation
    B. Managed care HMO/PPO
    C. Automobile insurance
    D. All of the above

34. In record keeping for tax time it is important to
    A. Record what activity you do hour by hour
    B. Keep track of the names of clients
    C. Keep track of automobile business mileage in a ledger
    D. None of the above

35. If you are in business for yourself it is important to
    A. Spend the money as you please and use December for taxes
    B. Save money for taxes
    C. Belong to a professional association
    D. Invest your money in the stock market

36. All of the following are retirement plans to help manage your money except
    A. Roth IRA
    B. IRA
    C. NCTMB

D. 401(K)

37. Business activities directed toward promoting and increasing business are called
   A. Assets
   B. Reputation
   C. Marketing
   D. Goals

38. Developing personal and professional contacts for the purpose of giving and receiving support and sharing information is called
   A. Hotline
   B. Networking
   C. Advertising
   D. Promotions

39. A business that has stockholders is called a
   A. Sole proprietorship
   B. Partnership
   C. Corporation
   D. Subsidiary

40. Professional arrangement(s) are available to massage therapists or bodyworkers who work with clients for insurance reimbursement
   A. The physician pays the therapist
   B. The client pays the therapist
   C. The insurance company pays the therapist
   D. All of the above

41. The current status of insurance reimbursement for massage is (are)
   A. Licensed massage therapists are the only ones to receive payment
   B. Nurses are the only ones to receive payment
   C. Massage has to be done in the doctor's office
   D. None of the above

42. The costs of education are deductible if
   A. They improve your professional skills
   B. You are training in a new field
   C. You are paying for massage school
   D. They are to meet minimal professional requirements

43. The insurance that covers costs of injuries occurring on your property and any resulting litigation is called
   A. Disability
   B. Liability
   C. Homeowner's
   D. Comprehensive

44. To qualify as a deductible home office
   A. It must be used exclusively for massage
   B. It must be used regularly in your practice
   C. You can deduct a portion of all living expenses
   D. It can be used as a den or bedroom as well

45. Massage therapists that are self-employed
   A. Have a business profit if after deductions have a profit
   B. Report on IRS form Schedule C
   C. Pay self-employment tax and income tax
   D. All of the above

46. In a personal service business, hygiene and safety are especially important to
   A. The client
   B. The facility
   C. The practitioner
   D. Everyone concerned

47. Business and personal deductions of income tax include all but the following
   A. Cost of supplies
   B. They reduce the total taxes you have to pay
   C. Professional association dues
   D. The cost of a car

48. A taxpayer identification number can be defined as
   A. A number given by IRS form SS-4
   B. A social security number
   C. A pin number chosen and submitted to IRS
   D. A and B

49. It is important for the massage practitioner to know the difference between sensuality and
    A. Sensitivity
    B. Sexuality
    C. Common sense
    D. Sympathy

50. City or municipal governments have the legal power
    A. To require fingerprints
    B. To decide what businesses can operate in the city
    C. To require a physician's clearance of communicable disease
    D. All of the above

51. When you consider opening an office, start up costs include
    A. Massage table, phone, rent, ads, music, sheets
    B. Massage table only
    C. Business cards, phone, and table
    D. A cost of $500

52. The ability to set positive goals and put forth the energy and effort required to achieve them is
    A. Self-motivation
    B. Self-preservation
    C. Self-indulgence
    D. Selfishness

53. Business enterprises for profit entities include all but the following
    A. Limited liability company
    B. Proprietorships
    C. Membership or trust
    D. Corporations

54. If you have a business name you must register it with
    A. IRS
    B. City or state clerk's office

C. AMTA
    D. All of the above

55. Keep your knowledge current by
    A. Attending seminars
    B. Reading trade journals
    C. Joining professional associations
    D. All of the above

56. To practice good ethics is to be concerned about the welfare of the public and individual clients, as well as your personal and professional
    A. Health
    B. Reputation
    C. Clothing
    D. Lifestyle

57. A well-written business card can be used for
    A. Referrals
    B. Advertising
    C. Promotional discount
    D. All of the above

58. Developing business relationships with people who are also promoting a business is called
    A. Referral
    B. Volunteerism
    C. Networking
    D. A partnership

59. An important part of ethics is to keep client communications
    A. Repeated
    B. Confidential
    C. Written down
    D. Recorded

60. A good business practice to prevent burnout is (are)
    A. Take a vacation or time off
    B. Get a massage for yourself

C. Exercise

D. All of the above

61. Which of the following types of insurance provides you with income in the event that you cannot work due to illness or injury?

A. Professional liability

B. General liability

C. Business personal property

D. Disability insurance

62. Confidentiality of your client's records is required for many reasons. The primary reason is

A. To protect yourself if sued by the client

B. To ensure adequate information for insurance billing purposes

C. Professional ethics

D. You were told to do so by your instructor

63. Important business resources include a variety of business and civic organizations such as the

A. Public library

B. Service Core of Retired Executives (SCORE)

C. Small Business Association

D. All are important resources

64. You are self-employed. How often do you have to make estimated tax payments?

A. Once a month

B. Annually, before December 31 of the tax year

C. You do not; just pay your taxes before April 15 when the return is due

D. Quarterly

65. A massage therapist can get professional liability insurance from

A. Prudential Insurance Company

B. American Massage Therapy Association (AMTA)

C. U.S. Health Care

D. All of the above

1.

D. Client-practitioner agreement and policy statements are important to inform the client and protect the therapist. (*Fritz, p. 170*)

2.

D. When you are screening a client, always have ready questions to ask as well as an understanding of expectations of client or special needs. Being prepared helps the conversation and leaves the client with a sense of professionalism. (*Sohnen-Moe, p. 229*)

3.

D. SOAP charting is an efficient, effective way to document all types of healthcare treatment through a subjective and objective assessment and plan for the client. (*Thompson, p. 7*)

4.

D. When a massage therapist is confronted with obscene calls it is always best to be as professional as possible and explain the services of your business. (*Sohnen-Moe, p. 229*)

5.

D. Many massage therapists have difficulty and fail in their new business due to burnout, lack of funds, or lack of marketing skills. (*Fritz, pp. 151–155*)

6.

D. Communication on the phone is a way of creating an invisible impression to a potential client. It is essential to be as polite and professional as possible. (*Sohnen-Moe, p. 227*)

7.

B. A client should always be referred to another health practitioner if the treatment required goes beyond massage. (*Beck, p. 295*)

8.

D. The information in a contract should reflect the specific nature of your business and goals to prevent legal conflict. (*Sohnen-Moe, p. 140*)

9.

C. All independent contractors supply their own materials and equipment and are paid for their service one time without expecting any expenses to be paid. (*Sohnen-Moe, p. 139*)

10.

C. Reviewing accurate records prior to massage establishes confidence and trust on the part of the client. (*Beck, p. 302*)

11.

D. An employee is trained and paid regularly by the company to which they provide a service. IRS outlines these and other factors that determine the status of an employer. (*Sohnen-Moe, p. 139*)

12.

D. All personal information regarding a client should be kept in a secure place and confidential. (*Beck, p. 302*)

13.

D. Ethical concerns of massage therapists include sexual misconduct, practicing beyond your scope, poor advertising, misleading claims of curative abilities, and more. (*Sohnen-Moe, p. 62*)

14.

D. All massage therapists should follow the code of ethics concerning respect, integrity, and caring after obtaining national certification. (*Fritz, p. 38*)

15.

D. It is not ethical to charge prices that are only for the wealthy. In fact it is ethical to provide a sliding scale when necessary. (*Sohnen-Moe, p. 65*)

16.

D. Many consultants are available when opening a business including an attorney, the Small Business Administration (SBA), an accountant, and Chamber of Commerce. (*Fritz, p. 150*)

17.

D. The capitalized earnings, assets, cash flow, and present value and future earnings all are considered as methods for pricing a business. (*Sohnen-Moe, p. 206*)

18.

D. Violating massage Rules of Conduct can result in a warning, suspension, or revocation of license. (*Beck, p. 23*)

19.
D. Good communication between therapist and client can ensure client return, referrals, and effective therapeutic sessions. (*Sohnen-Moe, p.217*)

20.
D. Business expenses include the costs of license, insurance, cards, linens, professional clothes, and memberships. (*Sohnen-Moe, p. 84*)

21.
D. Documenting work and keeping a client file ensures a permanent record for IRS, client needs, and finances. (*Sohnen-Moe, p. 231*)

22.
D. Client files document all the work you have done for your use and for the IRS. (*Sohnen-Moe, p. 80*)

23.
D. Marketing includes business cards and brochures, publications, and presentations. (*Sohnen-Moe, pp. 114–117*)

24.
B. All-important information should be included on intake: name, address, phone, and physician. (*Sohnen-Moe, p. 209*)

25.
D. Business deductions include something that helps to develop or maintain your trade including equipment, rent, phone, and any professional fees. (*Ashley, p. 125*)

26.
D. The office location requires that you meet the local governmental requirements including application for new business, zoning, and fire and health inspection. (*Ashley, p. 55*)

27.
A. SOAP charting is an efficient and effective way to document all types of health care treatment. (*Thompson, p. 8*)

28.
B. The disbursement record comes from the checkbook, but columns separate each category of expenditure. (*Beck, p. 633*)

29.
A. Clients prefer to have a massage by someone who was referred rather than opening the yellow pages or responding to a flyer. (*Sohnen-Moe, p. 252*)

30.
C. Many massage therapists and bodyworkers are sole proprietors in which they are the only one in charge of the business. Renting a space or working from home can do this. (*Ashley, p. 34*)

31.
D. Insurance reimbursement requires a great deal of documentation, a physician referral, and a medical reason for doing the bodywork or massage. (*Ashley, p. 160*)

32.
B. This is a record of credit extended to clients. (*Beck, p. 637*)

33.
D. All kinds of insurance companies can reimburse for massage services including, workers compensation, managed care, liability, and automobile or group health insurance. (*Ashley, p. 163*)

34.
C. It is important to keep a record of car mileage related to business travel, keep receipts and cancelled checks and bills for tax time at the end of the year. (*Ashley, p. 167*)

35.
B. If you are self-employed the most difficult thing to do is put money aside in a savings account for year-end taxes. (*Ashley, p. 172*)

36.
C. NCTMB is the National Certification for Therapeutic Massage and Bodywork and it has no retirement plan. The IRA's and 401(K) are ways to save money tax-free. (*Ashley, p. 175*)

37.
C. Marketing is advertising, public relations, promotion, and client referrals. (*Beck, p. 642*)

38.
B. Networking enhances the extension of the business. (*Beck, p. 644*)

39.

C. Stockholders share in profits but are not legally responsible for the actions of the corporation. (*Beck, p. 622*)

40.

D. The client, physician, or insurance company can pay the massage therapist or bodyworker for reimbursement. Keep all records of billing for your records for insurance claims. (*Ashley, p. 159*)

41.

D. The variation of insurance policies, state laws, and licensing make the subject of insurance reimbursement very complicated; each case is individual. (*Ashley, p. 156*)

42.

A. You can deduct the cost of education, plus travel and meals if the education maintains or improves your professional skills or is required by law for keeping your professional status. (*Ashley, p. 135*)

43.

B. Liability insurance is part of a homeowner's policy but may not cover business-related occurrences. (*Beck, p. 626*)

44.

B. A home office must be used regularly, or exclusively for massage or business bookkeeping and cannot be used as another room, guest, or den. (*Ashley, p. 138*)

45.

D. Self-employed massage therapists always report on Schedule C for IRS and are subject to self-employment tax and income tax. Profits are calculated after business deductions. (*Ashley, p. 133*)

46.

D. Everyone concerned should be aware that safety and personal hygiene are essential to a healthy atmosphere. (*Beck, p. 287*)

47.

D. The cost of a car is not a tax deduction, only the travel expenses, gas, repair, and services. (*Ashley, p. 134*)

48.

D. A taxpayer number can be a social security number if you are a sole proprietor or have no employees or a taxpayer ID number applied for on IRS form SS-4. (*Ashley, p. 123*)

49.

B. Good ethics and professional conduct are required for a certified, licensed, or registered massage practitioner. (*Beck, p. 629*)

50.

D. Municipal governments have the right to restrict the businesses of massage therapy. They can require photo, fingerprints, educational certifications, or a physician clearance. (*Ashley, p. 122*)

51.

A. You will need many items to start an office, massage table, sheets, phone, rent and security, music, phone, brochures, and ads, all costing about $3,000. (*Ashley, p. 61*)

52.

A. Self-motivation means to make sacrifices when necessary. (*Beck, p. 30*)

53.

C. Membership and trusts are business entities that are not for profit and have compliance, tax, and liability consequences that require the assistance of attorneys and accountants. (*Salvo, p. 618*)

54.

B. When you give your business a name, trade name, or fictitious name you must file it with the city or state clerk's office to protect another business from using your name. (*Salvo, p. 620*)

55.

D. Learning about new aspects of the field of massage as a health science is important. (*Beck, p. 27*)

56.

B. Individual ethics become part of the professional code of ethics. (*Beck, p. 26*)

57.

D. A good business card can project who you are and what you do and can serve as an advertisement, referral card, or discount promotion. (*Salvo, p. 626*)

58.

C. Networking is a way to learn from others, such as the Chamber of Commerce, civic groups, professional memberships, massage conferences, and conventions. (*Salvo, p. 632*)

59.

B. Communicate in a confidential and professional manner without exposing personal matters. (*Beck, p. 27*)

60.

D. Burnout is being tired and unhappy with one's work. It includes boredom, depression, and lack of productivity, and decline in social skills and boundaries. Take time off or a vacation, read a novel, exercise, or get a massage. (*Salvo, p. 635*)

61.

D. Disability insurance protects your income if you become ill or have a prolonged injury. (*Salvo, p. 619*)

62.

C. Ethics are standards of acceptable and professional behavior. (*Beck, p. 629*)

63.

D. There are many business resources to use for information such as the SBA, public library, SCORE, Rotary Club, or Chamber of Commerce. (*Salvo, p. 632*)

64.

D. According to the IRS, self-employed individuals must make quarterly tax payments. (*Beck, p. 627*)

65.

B. Malpractice insurance is essential for a massage therapist. Professional organizations, such as AMTA, can provide liability protection. (*Fritz, p. 167*)

Comprehensive Simulated Exam

This simulated exam represents the content contained in the NCBTMB exam; that is, Human Anatomy, Physiology, and Kinesiology (27%); Clinical Pathology and Recognition of Various Conditions (20%); Massage Therapy and Bodywork Theory, Assessment, and Practice (41%); Professional Standards, Ethics, and Business Practices (12%).

Directions: Each of the numbered items or incomplete statements in this chapter is followed by answers or completions of the statement. Select the **ONE** lettered answer or completion that is **BEST** in each case. The maximum time to complete the exam is three hours.

1. The sequences and directions of Swedish massage strokes are most adapted to which anatomical or physiological situation?
   A. Muscle attachments
   B. Subcutaneous adipose tissue
   C. Autonomic nervous system
   D. Lymph drainage and venous return

2. Which **BEST** describes the effects of massage therapy?
   A. Increase venous and lymph flow
   B. Increase venous, decrease arterial flow
   C. Decrease venous and lymph flow
   D. Decrease venous, increase lymph flow

3. When massaging the thigh in the supine position, which muscle is involved?
   A. Hamstrings
   B. Quadriceps
   C. Gluteals
   D. Gastrocnemius

4. Massage is contraindicated for which of the following conditions?
   A. High blood pressure
   B. Constipation
   C. Keloid scar
   D. Adhesions

5. The iliopsoas flexes the hip because of its insertion on the
   A. Femur
   B. Greater trochanter
   C. Lesser trochanter
   D. Iliac crest

6. The tricuspid valve is found between the
   A. Right atrium and right ventricle
   B. Left ventricle and aorta
   C. Left ventricle and right ventricle
   D. Right atrium and left atrium

7. Which is a **TRUE** statement concerning Golgi tendon apparatus?
   A. Found in joint capsules
   B. Detects overall tension in tendon
   C. Originates in Purkinje fibers
   D. Activated by bagal reflex

8. Which muscles are adductors?
   A. Pectoralis and deltoid
   B. Pectoralis and latissimus dorsi
   C. Deltoid and latissimus dorsi
   D. Biceps and deltoids

9. Which muscle would be paralyzed if the sciatic nerve were severed?
   A. Trapezius
   B. Biceps femoris
   C. Gluteus maximus
   D. Erector spinae

10. Which most accurately describes the meridian system?
    A. Energy pathway moving randomly through the body
    B. Energy pathway moving superficially
    C. Energy pathway that doesn't affect organs
    D. 12 meridians and 2 vessels are pathways in which energy moves toward the surface of the body affecting organs

11. The best massage stroke to be used on a chronic sprain is
    A. Transverse friction
    B. Effleurage
    C. Pick-up
    D. Tapotement

12. Which condition is present when there is an injury of the ulnar nerve at the elbow?
    A. Inability to flex fingers fully
    B. Spasticity
    C. Flaccidity
    D. Spasms

13. The only joint where the axial skeleton articulates with the appendicular skeleton is
    A. Sternoclavicular

B. Glenohumeral

C. Sternoscapular

D. Scapularclavicular

14. What muscle is not part of the rotator cuff?

A. Supraspinatus

B. Infraspinatus

C. Teres major

D. Teres minor

15. Precision muscle testing, passive positioning, directional massage, and deep pressure are the physical techniques used in

A. SMB

B. TMJ

C. NMF

D. PBF

16. Acupuncture, *shiatsu,* polarity, and reflexology are examples of

A. Energetic manipulation

B. Behavioral barometer

C. Reactive circuits

D. Systematic massage

17. Lymph massage procedures begin at the

A. Tendons

B. Left thoracic lymph duct

C. Right thoracic lymph duct

D. Immune system

18. Cross-fiber massage must be applied in which direction to the fibers?

A. Horizontally

B. At right angles

C. Triangularly

D. Trapezoidally

19. Cold applied for therapeutic purposes is called

A. Cryptology

B. Cryotherapy

C. Ignorance

D. Cool ice

20. Thorough assessment of a client's condition reveals any

A. Lies

B. Weight gains

C. Credit gaps

D. Contraindications

21. Psychological benefits of massage include reduced tension and fatigue, calmer nerves, and

A. Therapeutics

B. Renewed energy

C. Improved circulation

D. Spasms

22. Friction, percussion, and vibration are techniques that

A. Stimulate

B. Relax

C. Strengthen

D. Weaken

23. The kneading technique in which the practitioner attempts to grasp tissue and gently lift and spread it out is called

A. Fulling

B. Pulling

C. Spreading

D. Nudging

24. Pressing one superficial layer of tissue against a deeper layer of tissue in order to flatten the deeper layer is called

A. Rolling

B. Spreading

C. Friction

D. Ironing

25. Nerve trunks and centers are sometimes chosen as sites for the application of

A. Rolling

B. Rocking

C. Pressure

D. Vibration

EXAM

26. A bath with a temperature of 85° F to 95° F is considered
    A. Cool
    B. Cold
    C. Tepid
    D. Hot

27. The procedure that uses a bouncing movement to improve the flow of lymph through the entire system is called lymphatic
    A. Bounce
    B. Sway
    C. Purging
    D. Pump manipulation

28. The attempt to bring the structure of the body into alignment around a central axis is called
    A. Structural integration
    B. Trauma
    C. Alignment
    D. Adjustment

29. Realignment of muscular and connective tissue and reshaping the body's physical posture is called
    A. Adjustment
    B. Centering
    C. Rolfing
    D. Posturing

30. A hyperirritable spot that is painful when compressed is called a (an)
    A. Trigger point
    B. Pain point
    C. Ampule
    D. Rolfing

31. Relieving soreness, tension, and stiffness benefits which system?
    A. Muscular
    B. Skeletal
    C. Respiratory
    D. Excretory

32. In which directions do Yin meridians flow?
    A. Superior to inferior
    B. Inferior to superior
    C. Lateral to medial
    D. Medial to lateral

33. Injuries that have a gradual onset or reoccur often are called
    A. Sprains
    B. Occupational
    C. Acute
    D. Chronic

34. A sudden involuntary contraction of a muscle is called a (an)
    A. Levator
    B. Proximal
    C. Isometric
    D. Spasm

35. An exercise in which you imagine turning a large wheel is called
    A. The wheel
    B. Grinding corn
    C. Grounding
    D. Centering

36. If a client's condition is outside the massage technician's scope of practice, the technician should
    A. Schedule extra sessions
    B. Refer the client to the proper professional
    C. Take more training
    D. Read textbooks

37. Describing how the organs or body parts function and relate to one another is the study of
    A. Physiology
    B. Histology
    C. Anatomy
    D. Pathology

38. The branch of biology concerned with the microscopic structure of living tissues is

A. Physiology
B. Histology
C. Anatomy
D. Pathology

39. Which meridians are innervated by massaging the medial thigh?
A. KI, LIV, SP
B. GB, ST, SP
C. LIV, ST, KI
D. GB, LIV, KI

40. A relaxing atmosphere for massage may be created with
A. Clothing
B. Music
C. Wall coverings
D. Carpet

41. Cardiac muscle tissue occurs only in the
A. Liver
B. Stomach
C. Heart
D. Mouth

42. Blood is an example of
A. Cardiac tissue
B. Connective tissue
C. Nerve tissue
D. Striated muscles

43. In anatomy, the sagittal plane divides the body into left and right parts by an imaginary line running
A. Vertically
B. Horizontally
C. Diagonally
D. Circularly

44. Cancer is a disease that can be spread through the
A. Genes
B. Lymphatic and blood system
C. Endocrine system

D. Digestive system

45. The general effects of percussion movements are to tone the muscles by
A. Vibration
B. Friction
C. Kneading
D. Hacking, cupping, slapping, beating

46. The Trager method uses movement exercises called
A. Gymnastics
B. Mentastics
C. Spirals
D. Athletics

47. Aligning major body segments through manipulation of connective tissue is the
A. Rolfing method
B. Traeger method
C. Palmer method
D. Reflexology method

48. The idea that the stimulation of particular body points affects other areas is called
A. Chiropractic
B. Reflexology
C. Rolfing
D. Touching

49. Applied kinesiology methods are designed to relieve stress on muscles and
A. Joints
B. Bones
C. Ligaments
D. Internal organs

50. To reduce adhesions and fibrosis, which movement is used?
A. Cross-fiber friction
B. Wringing
C. Pressing
D. Squeezing

51. Massage is not performed on an area that is
    A. Bleeding
    B. Swollen
    C. Burned
    D. All of the above

52. The tendino-muscle channels of the lung pass through muscles of the chest and arm that include
    A. Pectorals
    B. Biceps brachii
    C. Diaphragm
    D. All of the above

53. Severe strain of the trapezius and deltoid muscles is called
    A. Racquetball shoulder
    B. Tennis elbow
    C. Skier's snap
    D. Bowler's break

54. Overstretching of the gracilis and adductor muscle on the inner thigh results from
    A. Soccer
    B. Tennis
    C. Horseback riding
    D. Bowling

55. Severe varicose veins is a (an) _____ for massage.
    A. Indication
    B. Circulation
    C. Embolus
    D. Contraindication

56. A survivor of abuse can benefit from massage by
    A. Feeling a sense of safeness
    B. Releasing or letting go some of the abuse
    C. Retrieving memory
    D. All of the above

57. Which meridian is lateral to the midsagittal line of the posterior cervical vertebrae?
    A. Governing vessel
    B. Triple warmer
    C. Stomach
    D. Bladder

58. What forms the outer layer of the anterior and lateral abdominal wall?
    A. Rectus abdominis
    B. Transversalis
    C. Serratus anterior
    D. External oblique

59. The primary flexor of the distal phalange of the fingers is
    A. Flexor carpi ulnaris
    B. Pollices longus
    C. Flexor digitorum profundus
    D. Flexor carpi radialis

60. A basic pattern of energy for the stomach channel is
    A. 7 AM to 9 AM
    B. 7 PM to 9 PM
    C. 3 AM to 5 AM
    D. 3 PM to 5 PM

61. Sciatic nerve damage diminishes ability to
    A. Flex the hip
    B. Flex the knee
    C. Adduct the hip
    D. Abduct the hip

62. Deep strokes and kneading techniques can cause an increase in
    A. Vasoconstriction
    B. Blood flow
    C. Diastolic arterial pressure
    D. Systolic arterial pressure

63. What **BEST** describes the technique of Rolfing?
    A. Reflex zone therapy

B. German massage

C. Structural integration

D. Connective tissue massage

64. Manipulation of the occipital regions of the neck primarily affects

A. HT and BL meridians

B. CO and KI meridians

C. BL and GB meridians

D. ST and SP meridians

65. Facial paralysis is due to a lesion in which cranial nerve?

A. III

B. VI

C. VII

D. VIII

66. Which muscle elevates and depresses the scapula?

A. Trapezius

B. Latissimus dorsi

C. Rhomboids

D. All of the above

67. With the elbow flexed, which muscle supinates the palm?

A. Pronator

B. Supinator

C. Quadrator

D. Brachialis

68. Deep friction massage works **BEST** if it is applied

A. Directly over problem area

B. Proximal to problem area

C. Distal to problem area

D. Around the problem area

69. The cupping technique is **BEST** suited for

A. Acute bronchitis

B. Cancer of the lungs

C. Bronchiectasis

D. Acute tracheitis

70. The last step in clot formation is

A. Prothrombin to thrombin

B. Fibrinogen to fibrin

C. Platelet formation

D. Tissue trauma

71. The exchange of O_2 and CO_2 takes place in the

A. Alveoli

B. Bronchi

C. Bronchioles

D. Pleural cavity

72. The temperature range for hot immersion baths is **BEST** at

A. 85° F–95° F

B. 100° F–110° F

C. 125° F–150° F

D. 130° F–140° F

73. To treat the seventh cranial palsy (Bell's palsy), brisk friction kneading should be done

A. From the mandible to hairline vertically

B. From the hairline to mandible

C. Transversely with both hands

D. Not at all

74. The therapeutic benefit of friction is

A. Local hyperemia

B. Lymphatic drainage

C. Tonification

D. None of the above

75. In which directions do Yin meridians flow?

A. Superior to inferior

B. Inferior to superior

C. Lateral to medial

D. Medial to lateral

76. The best massage to use on a chronic sprain is

A. Effleurage

B. Pick-up

C. Transverse friction

D. Vibration

77. Which is a band of strong, fibrous tissue that connects the articular ends of bones and binds them together?
    A. Membrane
    B. Fascia
    C. Cancellous tissue
    D. Ligament

78. Which stroke most often begins and ends a massage?
    A. Effleurage
    B. Petrissage
    C. Friction
    D. Vibration

79. What is the first primary consideration before beginning massage treatment?
    A. Make sure the client is comfortable
    B. Make sure no jewelry is being worn
    C. Wash hands thoroughly
    D. Determine if contraindications are present

80. How should you vary massage treatment with the age of the patient?
    A. Progressively with increased age
    B. Shorter with increased age
    C. Shorter for very old and very young
    D. The same for any age

81. How should pressure be administered during effleurage?
    A. Even
    B. Heavy decreasing to light
    C. Intermittent
    D. Light to heavy

82. In oriental theory, Yin energy flows
    A. Anterior to posterior
    B. Dorsal to ventral
    C. Inferior to superior
    D. Superior to inferior

83. Massage can relieve pain without the use of
    A. Imagery
    B. Stimulation
    C. Drugs, alcohol, or narcotics
    D. Endorphins

84. Yoga is a form of meditation for
    A. Good appetite
    B. Muscle balance and relaxation
    C. Dancing
    D. Religion

85. In which massage technique should the fingers move tissue under the skin but not the skin itself?
    A. Tapotement
    B. Effleurage
    C. Vibration
    D. Friction

86. For which type of tissue is vibration the most unsuitable?
    A. Major nerve course
    B. Muscle origins
    C. Bony prominences
    D. Skeletal muscle

87. Hot compresses used immediately after injury do **NOT**
    A. increase blood flow
    B. reduce muscle spasm
    C. reduce swelling
    D. relieve pain

88. Which is the first step in beginning massage treatment?
    A. Apply lubricant
    B. Effleurage
    C. Determine contraindications
    D. Diagnose the patient

89. When giving CPR to a 6-year-old child, you use the
    A. Heel of one hand

B. Heel of two hands

C. Fingers of one hand

D. Fingers of two hands

90. The popliteus muscle of the leg
    A. Adducts
    B. Extends
    C. Plantar flexes the ankle
    D. Medially rotates the tibia

91. First aid for acute soft tissue injuries involves RICE, which means
    A. Ice
    B. Rest and elevation
    C. Compression
    D. All of the above

92. Massage treatment of the chest should **NEVER** be done over the
    A. Ribs
    B. Heart
    C. Female nipples
    D. All of the above

93. Which aims most specifically to passively stretch muscle?
    A. Effleurage
    B. Friction
    C. Petrissage
    D. Tapotement

94. Massage benefits lymph flow **BEST** when strokes are
    A. Away from the heart
    B. Toward the heart
    C. Heavy in both directions
    D. In certain local areas

95. Shin-splint syndrome affects the
    A. Lateral malleolus
    B. Periosteum around the tibia
    C. Fibula
    D. All of the above

96. The thoracic duct drains the
    A. Entire body below the ribs
    B. Head, neck, chest, left limbs
    C. Largest lymph drainage of the body
    D. All are true

97. Which muscle is innervated by the axillary nerve?
    A. Deltoid
    B. Brachial
    C. Pectoralis major
    D. None of the above

98. Which is best to prevent adhesions in muscle tissue?
    A. Friction and effleurage
    B. Friction and petrissage
    C. Friction and tapotement
    D. Friction only

99. Petrissage beginning just distal to the medial condyle and moving proximal to the gluteal fold affects what muscles?
    A. Anterior adductors
    B. Medial hamstrings
    C. Quadriceps
    D. Deltoids

100. In tapping a large area of the body, which massage maneuver is used?
    A. Percussion
    B. Friction
    C. Effleurage
    D. Petrissage

101. Which condition is always a contraindication for massage?
    A. Muscle spasm
    B. Phlebitis
    C. Rheumatoid arthritis
    D. Edema

102. The main purpose of deep transverse friction is to
  A. Separate muscle fibers
  B. Lengthen muscle
  C. Shorten muscle fibers
  D. Minimize pain

103. Adult body temperature is higher than normal at
  A. 37° C
  B. 98° F
  C. 98.6° F
  D. 39° C

104. The triple warmer controls
  A. Assimilation, digestion, elimination
  B. Assimilation, digestion, skin temperature regulation
  C. Digestion, elimination, skin temperature regulation
  D. Elimination, digestion, nervous system

105. What plantarflexes and everts the foot?
  A. Tibialis anterior
  B. Gastrocnemius
  C. Plantaris
  D. Peroneus longus

106. Which muscle inserts into the iliotibial band?
  A. Gluteus maximus
  B. Quadratus femoris
  C. Gluteus medius
  D. Tensor fascia latae

107. Contraindications for hydrotherapy include all of the following EXCEPT
  A. Kidney infection
  B. Cold
  C. High or low blood pressure
  D. Skin infection

108. Massage therapy is used in pain management for
  A. Cardiac and terminal cancer patients
  B. Posttrauma patients
  C. Postsurgical patients
  D. All of the above

109. Connective tissue massage (CTM) is a useful technique for
  A. Preparing for surgery
  B. Psychoemotional status
  C. Loosening tissue following surgery or trauma
  D. Controlling pain

110. The primary physiological effect of massage therapy includes all of the following EXCEPT
  A. Delivery of oxygen to cells
  B. Clearance of metabolic waste and by-product of tissue damage
  C. Increase in blood and lymph circulation
  D. Increase in interstitial fluid and hydrostatic pressure

111. Vodder's manual lymph drainage (MLD) was developed for the specific purpose of
  A. Promoting lymph flow from tissue
  B. Eliminating the pneumatic cuff
  C. Decreasing urine output
  D. Increasing erythrocyte count

112. Fibrosis, the formation of abnormal collagenous connective tissue, is best treated by
  A. Deep friction massage
  B. Passive movements
  C. Kneading
  D. All of the above

113. The analgesic effect of ice massage is to
  A. Block pain-impulse conduction
  B. Reroute pain
  C. Decrease ROM
  D. Eliminate pain

114. Business expenses can include
  A. Business cards and advertising

B. Professional clothes and linens

C. License, insurance, and memberships

D. All of the above

115. Client files are important because

A. The Internal Revenue Service requires record keeping

B. Practitioner's must keep well informed of client's needs

C. You have documented your "work" on clients

D. All of the above

116. Good bookkeeping for healing arts professionals can

A. Eliminate tracking sheets

B. Decrease bank statements

C. Increase petty cash funds

D. Increase legitimate tax deductions

117. If you are a self-employed massage therapist, you must file

A. No returns

B. Only Schedule C—Profit or Loss form

C. Form 1040 and Social Security Self-Employment Tax form

D. B and C

118. Beneficial techniques to market professional skills include

A. Publications and presentations

B. Business cards and brochures

C. Donation of services

D. All of the above

119. Good client records should include

A. Intake form

B. Intake, health information, treatment, and session notes

C. Client history

D. Payments received

120. A typical client intake form should include

A. Name and address

B. Name, address, occupation, physician, emergency number

C. Name, phone, hobbies

D. Name, marital status, children

121. Massage can be effective in all of the following **EXCEPT**

A. Facilitating rehabilitation

B. Inhibiting a psychological effect

C. Preparing healthy muscles for strenuous activity

D. Enhancing the healing process

122. The purpose of a lubricant when massaging is to

A. Keep the body greasy

B. Prevent blisters from forming

C. Cleanse the body for relaxation

D. Avoid uncomfortable friction between the therapist's hand and the patient's skin

123. The reflex effects of massage are the stimulation of

A. Motor neurons

B. Sensory receptors of skin and subcutaneous tissues

C. Synovial fluid at each joint

D. Chemotransmitter

124. The benefits of massage to the skin, with the aim of returning it to normal function, include

A. Slowing metabolism

B. Removal of excretory products and dead skin

C. Decrease of hair growth

D. Preventing scar tissue from forming

125. Endorphins, which act like morphine for pain relief, are released from the

A. ANS

B. Midbrain

C. Limbic system and brain stem

D. CNS

126. The purpose of effleurage in massage is
  A. Relaxation
  B. ROM
  C. To search for spasms and spread lubricant
  D. To apply pressure to the spine

127. The kneading motion of petrissage serves to "milk" the muscle and
  A. Remove waste products
  B. Assist abnormal inactivity
  C. Assist venous return
  D. All of the above

128. The Chinese consider the lung as the delicate organ because
  A. It is a delicate tissue
  B. It is the first organ to be injured by negative substances
  C. It cannot work without the heart
  D. All of the above

129. Which term means "on the opposite side of the body?"
  A. Contralateral
  B. Distal
  C. Intermediate
  D. Proximal

130. Which element is needed for clotting and muscle contraction, and contributes to the hardness of teeth and bone?
  A. Calcium
  B. Hydrogen
  C. Iron
  D. Nitrogen

131. Jin Shin Do is an oriental therapy that is
  A. Preventative rather than symptomatic in nature
  B. To strengthen our absorption of life energy
  C. Acupressure with breathing and meditation

D. All of the above

132. An energy balancing therapy that attempts to remove blockages and bring healing energy to the problem areas is called
  A. Reflexology
  B. Therapeutic touch
  C. Amma therapy
  D. Myofascial release

133. A second-degree burn is characterized by
  A. Involvement of the entire epidermis and possibly some of the dermis
  B. No loss of skin functions
  C. Damage to most hair follicles and sweat glands
  D. Never scarring

134. Which of the following is defined as the degeneration of cartilage that allows the bony ends to touch and that is usually associated with the elderly?
  A. Osteoarthritis
  B. Osteogenic sarcoma
  C. Osteomyelitis
  D. Osteopenia

135. The Amma therapy is a full-body manipulation of the coetaneous regions, twelve organ channels, governing and conception vessels as well as
  A. Tendino-muscle channels
  B. TS points
  C. Yin-yang
  D. Qi of the heaven

136. Which of the following joint classifications is described as freely movable?
  A. Amphiarthrosis
  B. Cartilaginous
  C. Diarthrosis
  D. Fibrous

137. Which facial muscle inserts into the mandible, angles of the mouth, and skin of the lower face?
    A. Buccinator
    B. Depressor labii inferior
    C. Levator labii superioris
    D. Platysma

138. What is the spinal nerve contribution that composes the brachial plexus?
    A. C_1–C_4; T_1
    B. C_5–C_8; T_1
    C. C_7–C_8; T_1
    D. T_2–T_{12}; L_1

139. The sciatic nerve is actually two nerves. Which nerves comprise the sciatic nerve?
    A. Common peroneal and pudendal
    B. Tibial and medial plantars
    C. Medial and lateral plantars
    D. Common peroneal and tibial

140. Which of the following is the major muscle involved in crossing one's leg?
    A. Gastrocnemius
    B. Rectus femoris
    C. Sartorius
    D. Semimembranosus

141. The cerebellum
    A. Functions to maintain proper posture and equilibrium
    B. Receives input from the motor cortex and basal ganglia
    C. Receives input from proprioceptors in joints and muscles
    D. Has all of the above characteristics

142. A critical principle of holistic health is that the mind and body
    A. Are separate from the organs
    B. Function independently
    C. Is seen as a single entity

    D. Forces the healing process

143. The blood type that is termed the "universal donor" is
    A. O
    B. A
    C. B
    D. AB

144. The most numerous formed element in the blood is the
    A. Thrombocyte
    B. Leukocyte
    C. Erythrocyte
    D. Monocyte

145. Which of the following is characteristic of the sympathetic nervous system?
    A. Decreased heart rate
    B. Constricted pupils
    C. Splitting of glycogen to glucose in the liver
    D. Constriction of the bronchioles

146. The Ki flow through the meridians is the
    A. Hara breathing meditation
    B. Blockage
    C. Universal life energy
    D. Spirit

147. Which point(s) should be checked while practicing?
    A. Is the stance of good body positioning and height?
    B. Is the patient comfortable and relaxed?
    C. Is the pressure even throughout each stroke?
    D. All of the above

148. Variations of effleurage include
    A. Knuckling and stroking
    B. Backstroke and friction
    C. Pressure and brushing
    D. Wide angling and stroking

149. Variations of petrissage include
    A. One-handed petrissage
    B. Open and closed "C" position
    C. "V" hand position
    D. All of the above

150. Adhesions of a well-healed scar can be broken down between skin tissue by applying
    A. Vibration
    B. Petrissage
    C. Friction
    D. Effleurage

Comprehensive Simulated Exam

Answer Key

1. **D**	18. **B**	35. **A**	52. **D**
2. **A**	19. **B**	36. **B**	53. **A**
3. **B**	20. **D**	37. **A**	54. **C**
4. **A**	21. **B**	38. **B**	55. **D**
5. **C**	22. **A**	39. **A**	56. **D**
6. **A**	23. **A**	40. **B**	57. **D**
7. **B**	24. **C**	41. **C**	58. **D**
8. **B**	25. **D**	42. **C**	59. **C**
9. **B**	26. **C**	43. **A**	60. **A**
10. **D**	27. **D**	44. **B**	61. **B**
11. **A**	28. **A**	45. **D**	62. **B**
12. **C**	29. **C**	46. **B**	63. **C**
13. **A**	30. **A**	47. **A**	64. **C**
14. **C**	31. **A**	48. **B**	65. **C**
15. **A**	32. **B**	49. **D**	66. **A**
16. **A**	33. **D**	50. **A**	67. **B**
17. **C**	34. **D**	51. **D**	68. **D**

69. C	90. D	111. A	132. C
70. B	91. D	112. D	133. A
71. A	92. C	113. A	134. A
72. B	93. A	114. D	135. A
73. A	94. B	115. D	136. C
74. A	95. B	116. D	137. D
75. B	96. B	117. C	138. B
76. C	97. A	118. D	139. D
77. D	98. A	119. B	140. C
78. A	99. B	120. B	141. D
79. D	100. A	121. B	142. C
80. C	101. B	122. D	143. A
81. A	102. A	123. B	144. C
82. C	103. D	124. B	145. C
83. C	104. C	125. C	146. C
84. B	105. D	126. A	147. D
85. D	106. D	127. C	148. A
86. C	107. B	128. B	149. D
87. C	108. D	129. A	150. C
88. C	109. C	130. A	
89. A	110. D	131. D	

Figures

MERIDIANS

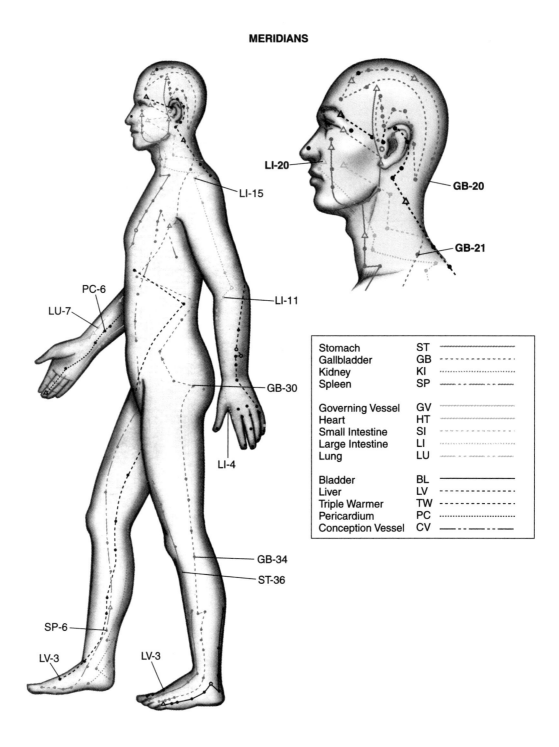

Stomach	ST
Gallbladder	GB
Kidney	KI
Spleen	SP
Governing Vessel	GV
Heart	HT
Small Intestine	SI
Large Intestine	LI
Lung	LU
Bladder	BL
Liver	LV
Triple Warmer	TW
Pericardium	PC
Conception Vessel	CV

Source: Tappan's Handbook of Healing Massage Techniques, 3/E by Tappan, F.M. and Benjamin, P.J. © 1998. Reprinted by permission of Pearson Education, Inc., Upper Saddle River, NJ.

MERIDIANS

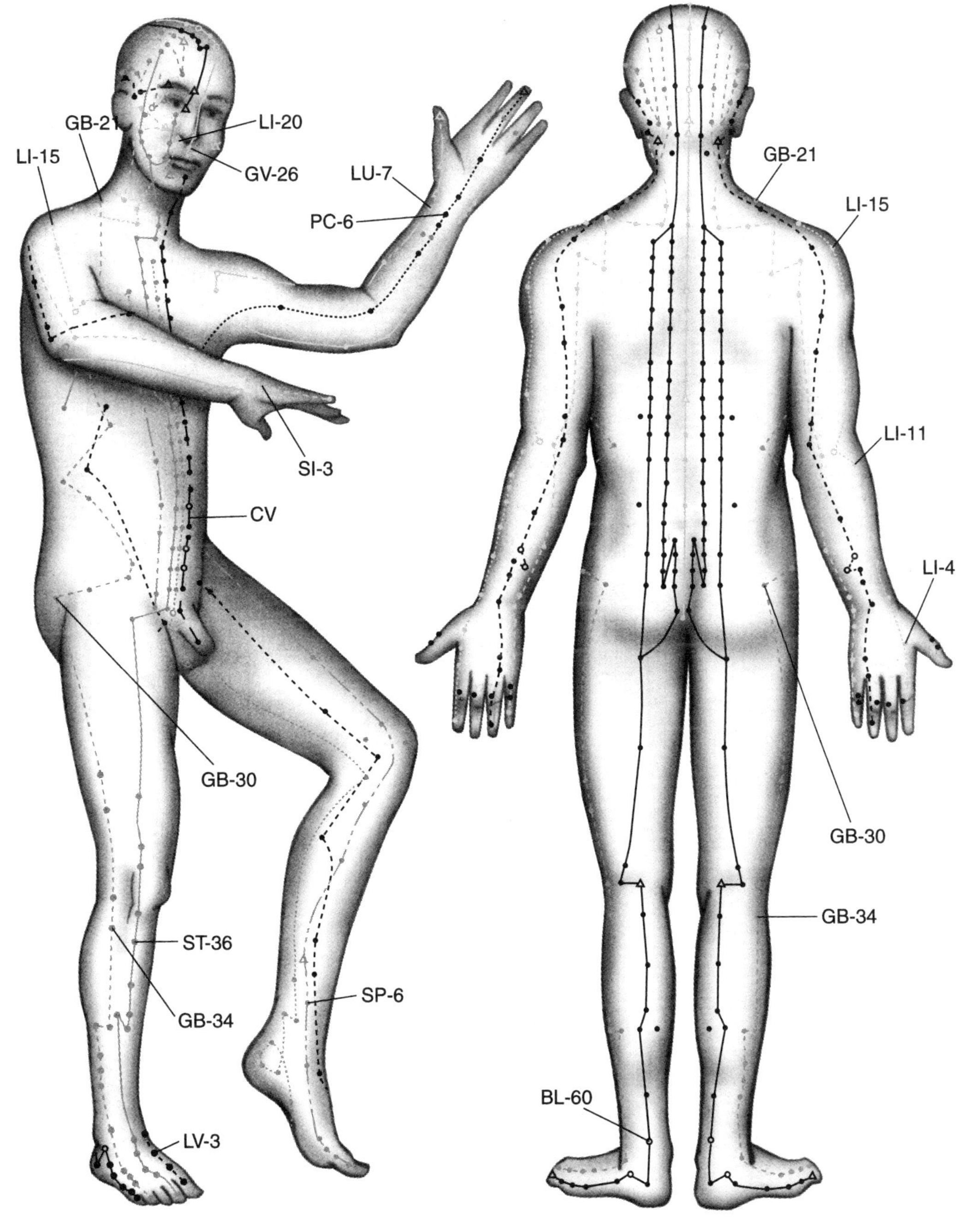
GB-21
LI-20
LI-15
GV-26
LU-7
PC-6
SI-3
CV
GB-30
ST-36
SP-6
GB-34
LV-3
GB-21
LI-15
LI-11
LI-4
GB-30
GB-34
BL-60

Source: Tappan's Handbook of Healing Massage Techniques, 3/E by Tappan, F.M. and Benjamin, P.J. © 1998. Reprinted by permission of Pearson Education Inc., Upper Saddle River, NJ.

ANTERIOR MUSCLES

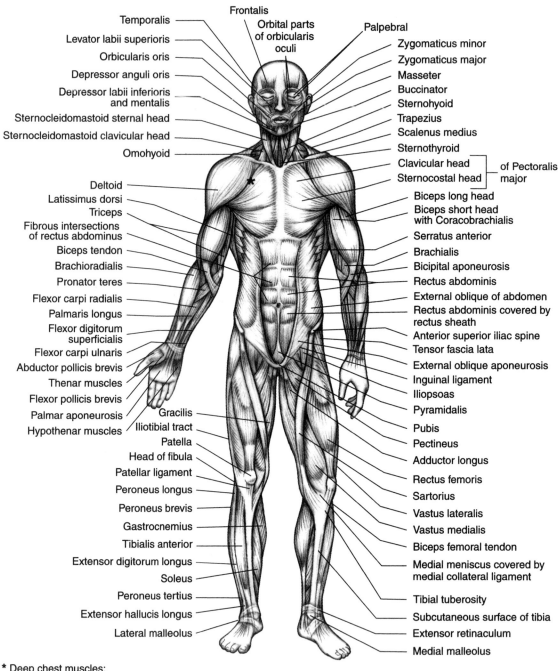

Temporalis
Levator labii superioris
Orbicularis oris
Depressor anguli oris
Depressor labii inferioris and mentalis
Sternocleidomastoid sternal head
Sternocleidomastoid clavicular head
Omohyoid

Frontalis
Orbital parts of orbicularis oculi

Palpebral
Zygomaticus minor
Zygomaticus major
Masseter
Buccinator
Sternohyoid
Trapezius
Scalenus medius
Sternothyroid
Clavicular head ⎤ of Pectoralis
Sternocostal head ⎦ major

Deltoid
Latissimus dorsi
Triceps
Fibrous intersections of rectus abdominus
Biceps tendon
Brachioradialis
Pronator teres
Flexor carpi radialis
Palmaris longus
Flexor digitorum superficialis
Flexor carpi ulnaris
Abductor pollicis brevis
Thenar muscles
Flexor pollicis brevis
Palmar aponeurosis
Hypothenar muscles

Gracilis
Iliotibial tract
Patella
Head of fibula
Patellar ligament
Peroneus longus
Peroneus brevis
Gastrocnemius
Tibialis anterior
Extensor digitorum longus
Soleus
Peroneus tertius
Extensor hallucis longus
Lateral malleolus

Biceps long head
Biceps short head with Coracobrachialis
Serratus anterior
Brachialis
Bicipital aponeurosis
Rectus abdominis
External oblique of abdomen
Rectus abdominis covered by rectus sheath
Anterior superior iliac spine
Tensor fascia lata
External oblique aponeurosis
Inguinal ligament
Iliopsoas
Pyramidalis
Pubis
Pectineus
Adductor longus
Rectus femoris
Sartorius
Vastus lateralis
Vastus medialis
Biceps femoral tendon
Medial meniscus covered by medial collateral ligament
Tibial tuberosity
Subcutaneous surface of tibia
Extensor retinaculum
Medial malleolus

* Deep chest muscles:
  • pectoralis minor
  • subscapularis

Source: Tappan's Handbook of Healing Massage Techniques, 3/E by Tappan, F.M. and Benjamin, P.J. © 1998. Reprinted by permission of Pearson Education, Inc., Upper Saddle River, NJ.

POSTERIOR MUSCLES

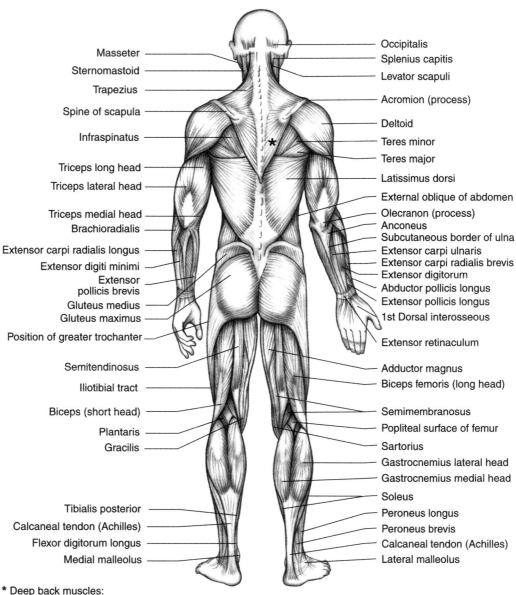

Masseter
Sternomastoid
Trapezius
Spine of scapula
Infraspinatus
Triceps long head
Triceps lateral head
Triceps medial head
Brachioradialis
Extensor carpi radialis longus
Extensor digiti minimi
Extensor pollicis brevis
Gluteus medius
Gluteus maximus
Position of greater trochanter
Semitendinosus
Iliotibial tract
Biceps (short head)
Plantaris
Gracilis
Tibialis posterior
Calcaneal tendon (Achilles)
Flexor digitorum longus
Medial malleolus

Occipitalis
Splenius capitis
Levator scapuli
Acromion (process)
Deltoid
Teres minor
Teres major
Latissimus dorsi
External oblique of abdomen
Olecranon (process)
Anconeus
Subcutaneous border of ulna
Extensor carpi ulnaris
Extensor carpi radialis brevis
Extensor digitorum
Abductor pollicis longus
Extensor pollicis longus
1st Dorsal interosseous
Extensor retinaculum
Adductor magnus
Biceps femoris (long head)
Semimembranosus
Popliteal surface of femur
Sartorius
Gastrocnemius lateral head
Gastrocnemius medial head
Soleus
Peroneus longus
Peroneus brevis
Calcaneal tendon (Achilles)
Lateral malleolus

* Deep back muscles:
  • erector spinae
  • multifidus
  • rhomboids
  • quadratus lumborum

Source: Tappan's Handbook of Healing Massage Techniques, 3/E by Tappan, F.M. and Benjamin, P.J. © 1998. Reprinted by permission of Pearson, Education, Inc., Upper Saddle River, NJ.

References

The following references or books have been used by the National Certification Board for Therapeutic Massage and Bodywork (NCTMB) for development of the Certifying Examination and have been used in preparation for review book content areas.

1. American Red Cross. *Standard First Aid.* St. Louis, MO: Mosby Lifeline, 1993.
2. Beck M. *The Theory and Practice of Therapeutic Massage.* Albany, NY: Milady Publishing Corporation, 1998.
3. Kapit W and Laurence E. *The Anatomy Coloring Book.* New York, NY: HarperCollins, 2001.
4. Sohnen-Moe C. *Business Master,* 3rd ed. Tucson, AZ: Sohnen-Moe Associates, 1997.
5. Tappan FM. *Healing Massage Technique: Holistic, Classic, and Emerging Methods.* Norwalk, CT: Appleton & Lange, 1998.
6. Thomas CL (ed). *Taber's Cyclopedic Medical Dictionary,* 16th ed. Philadelphia, PA: FA Davis, 1989.
7. Thompson CW and Floyd RT. *Manual of Structural Kinesiology,* 14th ed. St. Louis, MO: Times Mirror/Mosby College, 2001.
8. Tortora GJ and Grabowski SR. *Principles of Anatomy and Physiology,* 9th ed. New York: John Wiley & Sons, 2000.
9. Yates J. *A Physician's Guide to Therapeutic Massage.* Vancouver, BC: Massage Therapists' Association of British Columbia, 1990.

The following references have been added to expand the exam question resources to add non-Western techniques and holistic and touch therapy modalities and to increase business, ethics, and clinical pathology questions.

10. Ashley, M. *Massage: A Career at Your Fingertips,* 3rd ed. Brewster, NY: Enterprising Publishers, 1999.
11. Biel A. *Trail Guide to the Body.* Boulder, CO: Andrew Biel, 1997.
12. Chaitow L. *Muscle Energy Techniques.* New York: Churchill Livingston–Harcourt Brace, 1999.
13. Damjanov I. *Pathology for Health-Related Professions,* 2nd ed. Philadelphia, PA: WB Saunders–Harcourt Brace, 2000.
14. Fritz S. *Fundamentals of Therapeutic Massage.* St. Louis, MO: Mosby Lifeline, 2000.
15. Fritz S, Paholsky-Maison K and Grosenbach JM. *Mosby's Basic Science for Soft Tissue and Movement Therapies.* St Louis, MO: Mosby, 1999.
16. Hinkle CZ. *Fundamentals of Anatomy and Movement.* St. Louis, MO: Mosby, 1997.
17. Lundberg P. *The Book of Shiatsu.* New York, NY: Simon & Schuster, 1992.
18. Salvo SG. *Massage Therapy–Principles & Practices.* Philadelphia, PA: WB Saunders Co.–Harcourt Brace, 1999.
19. Sieg KW and Adams SP. *Illustrated Essentials of Musculoskeletal Anatomy,* 3rd ed. Gainesville, FL: Megabooks, 1996.

20. Sohn T. and R. *Amma Therapy: A Complete Textbook of Oriental Bodywork and Medical Principles.* Rochester, VT: Healing Arts Press, 1996.

21. Teaguarden, I. *Acupressure: Way of Health.* Tokyo and New York: Jin Shin Do Japan Publishers, 1995.

22. Thompson DL. *Hands Heal: Communication, Documentation, and Insurance Billing for Manual Therapists,* 2nd ed. Baltimore, MD: Lippincott Williams & Wilkins, 2002.

23. Thompson DL. *Hands Heal: Documentation for Massage Therapy.* Seattle, WA: Diana L. Thompson, 2002.

24. Travell JG and Simons DG. *Myofascial Pain and Dysfunction: The Trigger Point Manual Vol 1 & 2.* Baltimore, MD: Lippincott Williams & Wilkins, 2001.

25. Werner R and Benjamin BE. *A Massage Therapist Guide to Pathology.* Baltimore, MD: Williams & Wilkins, 1998.

26. Yates, J. *A Physician's Guide to Therapeutic Massage.* Vancouver, BC: Massage Therapists' Association of British Columbia, 1990.

Glossary

Abdominal – anterior trunk.

Abductors – moving of a part of the body away from the center of the body.

Absolute contraindications – those conditions that massage may be harmful and not indicated.

Acetylcholine – a chemical that mediates nerve activity to the skeletal muscles.

Acne vulgaris – an infection of the sebaceous glands and hair follicles, caused by bacteria.

Acquired immunodeficiency syndrome AIDS – a disease caused by the human immunodeficiency virus (HIV).

Active assisted stretching – stretching in which the client contracts the agonist to stretch the antagonist while outside forces assist the lengthening action.

Active resisted stretches or isometric movements – gentle resistance applied by the therapist while the client is actively engaging in the stretch.

Acupressure – a western term for a form of bodywork based on the meridian theory in which acupuncture points are pressed to stimulate the flow of energy or *Chi*.

Acupuncture – is the Chinese medical practice in which the skin is punctured with needles at specific points along the meridian channels or paths of energy.

Acute – conditions that last for a short time.

Addison's disease – partial or complete failure of adrenal functions, which can result from an autoimmune disease, local or general infection, or adrenal hemorrhage.

Adductors – muscles when flexed pull part of the body toward the body.

Adhesion – fibrous tissue that forms an abnormal union between two previously separate structures.

Agonist – muscle that is most responsible for causing desired joint action.

All or none response – when each individual muscle fiber, when sufficiently stimulated contracts to its fullest and in the absence of sufficient stimuli each muscle fiber relaxes to its fullest.

Allergies – hypersensitivity and overreaction to otherwise harmless agents.

Amma – a form of traditional Japanese massage using acupressure.

Amphiarthrotic joints – joints that are slightly moveable.

Anatomical position – standard body position. The body is erect and facing forward, arms are at the side, palms forward while feet are slightly apart, and toes pointing forward.

Anemia – decrease in red blood cells or decrease in the amount of functional hemoglobin in the blood, which decreases the oxygen-carrying capacity of the blood causing this condition.

Angina pectoris – chest pain, often caused by constriction of coronary arteries and myocardial anoxia (lack of oxygen in the heart muscle).

Ankylosing spondylitis – inflammatory disease causing calcification and fusion of the joints between the vertebrae and sacroiliac joint.

Anterior or ventral – the front of a structure.

Antiseptic – a substance that retards pathogenic growth and removes pathogenic organisms from tissue without destroying the tissue.

Apnea – spontaneous respiration is temporarily stopped or absent.

Aponeurosis – the attachment of skeletal muscle to bone, to another muscle, or to the skin by a broad, flat tendon.

Arrector pili – the muscles of the hair that allow them to stand upright.

Arteries – vessels that move blood away from the heart.

Arteriosclerosis – arteries narrowing due to the accumulation of lipid plaques in the walls, reducing blood flow.

Arthritis – chronic disease characterized by inflammation, swelling, and pain in the joints.

Asthma – a respiratory disorder characterized by difficulty in breathing, wheezing, coughing, and thick mucous production caused by inflammation of the bronchi.

Atrium – superior heart chambers that receive blood from the body through large veins.

Autoimmune diseases – a group of diseases, which are characterized by an alteration of immune functions. This is a result of an attack by the body's own immune system.

Axillary – armpit, the pyramid-shaped area formed by the underside of the anterior and posterior aspects of the shoulder.

Axon or efferent processes – a single cylindrical extension of the neural cell that transmits impulses away from the cell body.

Ball and socket joint – type of joint, which permits all movements and offers the greatest range of movement (e.g. the hip (iliofemoral joint) and shoulder (glenohumeral joint)). Also known as a *spheroid* or a *triaxial joint.*

Baroreceptors – pressure-sensitive receptor cells that affect blood pressure by sending impulses to the cardiac center and to the vasomotor center in the medulla oblongata.

Basement membrane – attaching surface of epithelial tissue.

Benign – condition that is not cancerous or life threatening.

Bindegewebsmassage – is a connective tissue massage believed to affect vascular and visceral reflexes.

Blood-brain barrier – a very selective semipermeable membrane that controls which substances are allowed into the brain.

Blood pressure – the pressure exerted by blood on an arterial wall during the contraction of the left ventricle.

Body mechanics – biomechanics, the use of proper body techniques to deliver massage therapy with the utmost efficiency and minimum trauma to the therapist.

Bone – the hardest and most solid of all connective tissue. Bone is made of compact tissue, a spongy cancellous tissue, collagenous fibers (for strength), and mineral salts (for hardness).

Bony landmarks – parts of bones that are used for reference to muscles (i.e., trochanter of the femur).

Boundaries – the space or limits we establish between others and ourselves regarding different aspects of our lives.

Bow stance – a foot stance used in massage therapy when performing any gliding strokes where length is important. The feet are placed on the floor in 90-degree angle, one pointing straight and one pointing toward the side.

Brachial – area in the upper arm, between the shoulder and the elbow.

Bradycardia – slow heart rate (fewer than 50–60 beats per minute).

Brain stem – the inferior part of the brain that contains three main structures: midbrain, pons, and medulla oblongata.

Bronchioles – smaller divisions of the bronchi.

Bronchitis – inflammation of the bronchial mucosa that causes the bronchial tubes to swell and extra mucus to be produced.

Buccal – pertaining to the cheek area.

Burnout – a condition of being tired of or unhappy with one's work. It does not discriminate against any race, sex, religion, or age. It is a condition that can be found in any profession.

Bursa – a saclike structure with a synovial membrane that contains synovial fluid.

Bursitis – acute or chronic inflammation of the bursae. Infection, trauma, disease, or excessive friction or pressure in the joint causes it.

Business personal property insurance – a type of insurance, which covers the cost of business property, such as a desk, massage table, chairs, and stereo equipment in your business location.

Calcitonin – decreases blood calcium and phosphorous by stimulating osteoblasts (bone-forming cells) to make bone matrix. This causes calcium and phosphorous to be deposited in the bones.

Capillaries – blood vessels with thin, permeable membranes for efficient gas exchange.

Capillary exchange – the system where nutrients and oxygen are provided to tissues and waste from cells is removed.

Carcinogen – cancer-causing agent.

Carpal tunnel syndrome – a painful repetitive strain injury of the hand and wrist caused by compression of the median nerve.

Cartilage – an avascular, tough, protective tissue capable of withstanding repeated stress. Since cartilage has no direct blood supply it is slow to heal.

Cell body, cyton, or soma – part of the neuron that contains the nucleus and other standard equipment (i.e., organelles) of the cell.

Centering – a mental, emotional, and physical state of the therapist that is calm, yet responsive.

Central nervous system – part of the nervous system that occupies a central or medial position in the body. It's primary purpose is to interpret incoming sensory information and with issuing instructions in the form of motor response. The major components of the CNS include the brain (i.e., cerebrum, cerebellum, diencephalons, brain stem), meninges, cerebrospinal fluid, and spinal cord.

Cerebellum – the cerebellum is concerned with muscle tone, coordinates skeletal muscles and balance (posture integration and equilibrium), and controls fine and gross motor movements. It is a cauliflower-shaped structure located posterior and inferior to the cerebrum.

Cerebral palsy – motor disorders resulting in muscular uncoordination and loss of muscle control.

Cerebrospinal fluid – a clear, colorless fluid circulating around the brain and spinal cord. It provides a medium for nutrient exchange and waste removal as well as shock absorbtion.

Cerebrum – the largest part of the brain that governs all higher function (i.e., language, memory, reasoning, and some aspects of personality).

Cervical – pertaining to the neck area.

Chemoreceptors – the activation of chemical stimuli by sensory receptors that detect smells, tastes, and chemistry changes in the blood.

Chronic – conditions that have a long duration, sometimes a lifetime.

Cirrhosis – a chronic degenerative disease of the liver in which the hepatic cells are destroyed and replaced with fibrous connective tissue, giving the liver a yellow-orange color.

Code of ethics – a guideline of moral principles that governs one's course of action.

Cold or ice immersion baths – a treatment of immersing the affected area in a container of icy/cold water. This method is convenient for feet and hands.

Collagen – an insoluble, fibrous protein that constitutes about 70 percent of the dermis and offers support to the nerves, blood vessels, hair follicles, and glands.

Compression massage – rhythmic pumping on a muscle belly to create a sustained increase in circulation and muscle relaxation.

Confidentiality – privileged information that may not be divulged to a third party without the client's permission.

Connective tissue – the most abundant and ubiquitous tissue of the body. Some connective tissue types serve as nutrient transport systems, some defend the body against disease, some possess clotting mechanisms, and others act as a supportive framework and provide protection for vital organs.

Contamination – air-borne, fluid-borne, direct contact of infectious or causative agents entering an organism. When an organism is contaminated, the next phase is infection.

Contract – a written agreement between two or more parties that outlines expectations, duties, and responsibilities which is enforceable by law.

Contracture – a condition of a joint, which is abnormal and usually permanent, where the muscle is fixed in a flexed position.

Contralateral – related to the opposite side of the body.

Contusion – an injury resulting from a blow to soft tissue. A contusion is commonly called a bruise. The discoloration comes from blood escaping from the blood vessels that were broken or damaged from the blow.

Cryotherapy – the application of cold on the body. The methods may include ice, icy water, frozen gel, or chemical cold packs.

Cushing's disease – a metabolic disorder caused by an overproduction of adrenocorticol steroids.

Cyriax, James – an osteopath from England who developed a system to test all joints to isolate lesions in the soft tissue.

Cytoplasmic organelles – small cellular structures that provide special functions such as reproduction, storage, and metabolism. Types of organelles are the nucleus, ribosomes, endoplasmic reticulum, Golgi apparatus, mitochondria, lysosomes, and centrioles.

Deltoid – large muscle of the upper arm that forms the curve of the shoulder and upper arm.

Dendrites or afferent processes – typically short, narrow and highly branched neural extensions that receive and transmit stimuli toward the cell body.

Dermis or corium – tissue under the epidermis that contains adipose tissue, many blood vessels, and nerve endings.

Diabetes mellitus – a group of conditions that lead to elevated blood glucose levels (hyperglycemia).

Diarthrotic joints – freely moveable joints allowing movement in more than one dimension. Also known as synovial joints.

Disability insurance – insurance that provides you with income even if you can not work due to illness or injury.

Disinfecting – the removal of pathogenic microorganisms from surfaces by a chemical or mechanical agent.

Dislocation – displacement of bones due to extreme force.

Distal – away from the point of reference, usually away from the midline or central point.

Diuretic – any substance that promotes the formation and excretion of urine.

Documentation – information that is recorded on paper.

Dorsal cavity – located on the back or posterior.

Draping – technique of covering the client with a drape during massage to promote warmth and professional atmosphere that satisfies the client's need for privacy and comfort.

Eczema – an acute or chronic superficial inflammation of the skin characterized by redness, watery discharge, crusting, scaling, itching, and burning.

Effleurage – a massage stroke of purposeful, gliding movements that follow the contour of the client's body.

Elastic cartilage – a soft and more pliable cartilage than hyaline or fibrocartilage that gives shape to the external nose and ears and to internal structures, such as the epiglottis and the auditory tubes.

Ellipsoidal joints – joints that are essentially a reduced ball and socket joint. Ellipsoidal joints allow flexion, extension, abduction, and adduction but rotation is not permitted (e.g., radiocarpal joints in the wrist). Also known as *condyloid* or *biaxial joints*.

Embolus – a blood clot, bubble of air, or any piece of debris transported by the bloodstream.

Emphysema – abnormal condition of the lungs in which there is over inflation of the alveoli of the lungs, leading to a breakdown of their walls and a decrease in respiratory function.

Endangerment sites – areas of the body that contain certain anatomical structures that are vulnerable to injury.

Endorphins – any natural protein in the brain that helps to reduce pain.

Epilepsy – neurological disorder characterized by convulsive seizures, impaired consciousness.

Epinephrine or adrenaline – an adrenal hormone that increases blood pressure by stimulating vasoconstriction, rather than affecting cardiac output.

Estrogen – female hormone that promotes the development of secondary sex characteristics in females.

Excursion – the distance traversed on the client's body or the length of a massage stroke.

Expiration or exhalation – a procedure that occurs when the diaphragm relaxes and ascends back up toward the thoracic cavity. Air is forced out of the lungs.

Extensor – a muscle that extends a joint.

External – nearest the outside of a body cavity.

Femoral or crural – pertaining to the femur or the thigh area, between the hip and the knee.

Fibrocartilage – of the three cartilage types the one with the greatest tensile strength. Fibrocartilage is found in the intervertebral disks, in the meniscus of the knee joint, and between the pubic bones (pubic symphysis).

Fibromyalgia – a chronic inflammatory disease that affects muscle and related connective tissue.

Fibrosis or scar formation – a process in which the original tissue type is replaced with a different kind of tissue. Fibrosis occurs when the damage is so severe that there are not enough healthy cells to reproduce the tissue required or when the damaged tissue does not have the ability to readily reproduce itself. The scar tissue formed by fibrosis is usually stronger than the original tissue.

Five elements – in Chinese medicine these are Water, Fire, Wood, Earth, and Metal that form a star.

Fixators or stabilizers – specialized synergists that stabilize the joint over which the prime mover exerts its action. This allows the prime mover to perform a motion more efficiently.

Flaccid – a condition where a muscle lacks normal tone and appears flattened rather than rounded.

Flexibility – the ability of the muscles, joints, and soft tissues to bend.

Flexor – a muscle that bends a joint.

Foot reflexology – a therapeutic system theory, which the entire body (organs, glands, and body parts) has reflex points located on the feet. By using applied pressure, one can release blockages around the corresponding body part and rebalance the entire body.

Fractures – a disruption in the structure of the bone. There are several types of fractures. A fracture is a break, chip, crack, or rupture of bone.

Free nerve endings or nociceptors – bare nerve endings that detect pain.

Friction – a brisk, often heat-producing compression stroke that may be delivered either superficially to the skin or to deeper tissue layers of muscle, depending upon the intention of the therapist.

Frontal or coronal plane – the plane passing through the body from side-to-side to create anterior (ventral) and posterior (dorsal) sections.

Fungus – a microorganism that requires an external carbon source; fungi reproduce by spore formation. Fungus growth is promoted by a warm and moist environment and includes molds and yeast.

Furunculous – a boil or an abscess caused by the staphylococcal bacteria resulting in necrosis (death) of a hair follicle.

Gait – the walking pattern.

Ganglion – a cluster of nerve cell bodies located in the peripheral nervous system.

General liability insurance – insurance that covers liability costs that are a result from bodily injury, property damage, and personal injury. Also referred to as *premise liability*.

Gliding joints – these joints permit movements limited to gliding in flexion, extension, abduction, and adduction (intercarpal and intertarsal joints). Also known as *arthrodia* or *biaxial joints*.

Gluteal – curve of the buttocks formed by the large gluteal muscles.

Golgi tendon organs – receptors that are stimulated by both tension and excessive stretch and are located at the musculotendinous boundary of skeletal muscles. These protective mechanism help to ensure that muscles do not become excessively stretched or do not contract too strongly and damage their tendons.

Gout – a disease in which a defect in uric acid metabolism causes acid and its salts to accumulate in the blood.

Hepatitis – inflammation of the liver.

Hernia – a protrusion of surrounding connective tissue or cavity wall of an organ or part of an organ.

Hinge joints – movements that are limited to flexion and extension (elbow and interphalangeal joints). Also known as *ginglymus* or *monoaxial joints*.

Homeostasis – a somewhat stable or balanced condition of the body's internal environment within a limited range.

Horse stance – positioning of feet during massage therapy when applying strokes that traverse relatively short distances such as petrissage and certain friction strokes. The feet are placed on the floor, toes pointing forward, and a little more than hip distance apart.

Hot pack – a means of applying moist heat for pain relief. Also known as *hydrocollator packs, fomentation packs, hot compresses,* and *hot dressings.*

Hydrotherapy – therapeutic use of water and complimentary agents (salt and soap) at temperatures no more than 8 degrees from normal body temperature. The water can be either cold or hot.

Hydrotherapy tubs or spas – immersion baths and whirlpool baths, where the water is treated to remain clean and sanitary for multiple use.

Hygiene – the principles of health maintenance.

Hyperemia – the noticeable reddened skin that results from increased blood flow.

Hypertension – elevated blood pressure; 140/90 mmHg is regarded as the threshold of hypertension and 160/95 is classified as serious hypertension.

Hypertrophy – increase in the size and diameter of muscle fibers without cell division.

Hypoglycemia – a condition of low blood sugar.

Hypoxia – a decrease in the amount of oxygen in the blood.

Ice massage – circular friction and cryotherapy.

Inferior or caudal – situated below or toward the tail end.

Inflammation – a protective mechanism with the purpose of stabilization and preparation for damaged tissue repair. It is the body's immediate reaction to soft tissue injury. The primary symptoms are localized heat, swelling, redness, pain and decreased range of motion.

Initial evaluation – the first report written from your SOAP notes.

Insertion – the muscle attachment undergoing the greatest movement.

Insulin – secreted by pancreatic beta cells, decreasing blood glucose levels by enhancing the uptake of glucose into the cells.

Interosseous membrane – a tough membrane that connects bones (ulna and radius) by attaching to their periosteum. Also known as interosseous ligament since it connects bone to bone.

Ischemia – a reduction of oxygenated blood to an organ or body part, marked by pain and tissue dysfunction.

Isometric contractions – increase in muscle contraction without change in muscle length or angle, no movement.

Isotonic or dynamic contractions – a contraction of the muscle where it changes length against resistance and movement occurs.

Jin Shin Do® – is a modern version of traditional Chinese Acupressure theory based on eight (8) *Strange Flows.* Iona Teeguarden developed it in 1970.

Kellogg, John Harvey (1852–1943) – an American dealing with health concerns. He wrote numerous articles and books on massage that brought its attention to the public.

Ki, Qi – energy along fourteen (14) meridians and 365 acupoints located throughout the body.

Kinesiology – the study of the body's muscles, joints, and their movements.

Kyphosis – is an abnormal convex curvature of the spine.

Lateral – located farthest away from the midline of the body.

Law of facilitation – a neurological law that states once an impulse has traveled a certain nerve pathway it tends to "imprint" or "facilitate" the pathway. Accordingly it will take the same path on future occasions.

Leukocytes – white blood cells or white corpuscles.

Ling, Pehr Henrik (1776–1839) – Swedish physiologist and gymnastics instructor. Known as the "father of Swedish massage." He developed his own system of medical gymnastics and exercise, known by different names–the Ling System, Swedish Movements, or the Swedish Movement Cure. An important part of the Ling System was a style known as Swedish Massage.

Local twitch response – an involuntary firing or twitching in muscle in response to the sensory stimulation on the trigger point.

Loose connective tissue – known as the packing material of the body. It attaches the skin to underlying structures, wraps and supports body cells, fills in the spaces between organs and muscles, and stabilizes them in their proper places.

Lordosis – is an abnormal concave curvature of the spine.

Lumbar – the area between the thorax and hips of the pelvis.

Lyme disease – the bacterium *Borrelia burgdorferi*, which is transmitted by a tick bite and causes a recurrent form of arthritis.

Lymph – the fluid of the lymph system.

Lymph nodes – structures located along lymph vessels that collect and filter lymph. They protect the body from unwanted invaders.

Malignant – a condition which can worsen and cause death if not treated.

Malignant melanomas – cancer of the melanocytes of the skin, which begin as raised dark lesions with irregular borders and appear uneven in color.

Massage – a systematic and scientific manipulation of the soft tissue for the purpose of improving and maintaining health. It can also be defined as organized intentional touch or therapeutic touch.

Mastication – process of chewing.

Mechanoreceptors – sensory receptors that respond to mechanical stimuli. They are sensitive to touch, pressure, vibration, stretching, muscular contraction, proprioception, sound, and equilibrium.

Medial – located more toward or near the midline of the body.

Meissner's corpuscles – receptors for light touch, responding to the actual movement, and the length of the movement. They monitor low-frequency vibration and adapt slowly.

Meningitis – an inflammation or infection of the meninges often characterized by a sudden severe headache, vertigo, stiff neck, and severe irritability.

Meridian – refers to the *Chi* energy that circulates through twelve channels passing through organs and the extremities.

Metabolic diseases – involves abnormal activities of cells and/or tissues (e.g., diabetes, cardiovascular conditions, and jaundice). Metabolic diseases are not contagious, but may have originated from a contagious disease, such as hepatitis, which can lead to jaundice or vice versa.

Metabolism – total of all chemical and physical processes that occur in an organism.

Metastasis – the spreading of cancerous cells to distant body parts usually by way of the bloodstream or lymphatic system.

Midsagittal or median plane – the plane that runs longitudinally or vertically, down the body, dividing the body into right and left sections. This plane creates a right lateral and left lateral portion of the body.

Modality – a broad term used to denote any technique, procedure, or product used to produce a positive response for the client.

Motor neurons – neurons responsible for carrying messages to muscles or glands.

Motor units – a single motor neuron and all it's associated skeletal muscle fibers. A single muscle is composed of many motor units.

Multiple sclerosis – the progressive destruction of myelin sheaths in the central nervous system.

Muscle cramp – acute, painful contraction of a muscle.

Muscle energy techniques (MET) – techniques of stretching, that use neurophysiological muscle reflexes to improve mobility of the joints.

Muscle fatigue – the inability of a muscle to contract even though it is still being stimulated.

Muscle or neuromuscular spindles – stretch sensitive receptors that monitor deviations in the length of a muscle and the rate of change.

Muscle spasm – an increase in muscle tension with or without shortening causing disability and pain.

Muscular atrophy – reduction of muscle size due to poor nutrition, lack of use, motor unit dysfunction, or lack of motor nerve impulses.

Muscular dystrophy – an inherited disease of the skeletal muscles that weakens and atrophies leading to increasing disability.

Myofascial – is a term for techniques aimed at restoring mobility in the body's fascia and softening connective tissue.

Myofilaments – bundles of smaller structures called actin and myosin that comprise a myofibril.

Negative feedback system – a method of the endocrine system that triggers the negative (opposite) response.

Nephrons – the filtering system of the kidneys that filters waste products from the blood.

Nerve – impulse carrying fibers connecting the brain and the spinal cord with other parts of the body.

Nerve compression – pressure against the nerve due to contact with hard tissue (bone or cartilage) also known as impingement.

Nerve entrapment – pressure against the nerve due to adjacent soft tissue (muscle, tendon, fascia, and ligaments) also known as entrapment neuropathy.

Networking – the development of business relationships with various groups of people with the similar views.

Neuroglia or glial cells – connective tissues that support, nourish, protect, insulate, and organize the neurons.

Neuromuscular or myoneural junction – fluid-filled space between nerve endings and muscle fibers.

Neuropathy – decrease or change in sensation in hands and feet.

Neurotransmitters – a collective term for a range of chemicals that facilitate, arouse, or inhibit the transmission of nerve impulses between synapses.

Nociceptor – receptors for detecting pain. Also known as *free nerve endings.*

Norepinephrine or noradrenaline – hormones that assist the body in maintaining the stress response. The effects are increased heart rate, blood pressure, and blood glucose levels, and dilation of the small passageways of the lungs.

Origin – the tendinous attachment of the muscle that is relatively fixed during the muscle's action.

Osteoarthritis – arthritis characterized by degeneration of cartilage in joints; more common in the elderly. Symptoms include pain after exercise or use, joint stiffness, and swelling.

Osteoporosis – decreased bone mass and increased susceptibility to fractures.

Outcome – the short or long term response of the client to therapy.

Pacinian's or laminated corpuscles – pressure sensitive receptors that respond to skin displacement and high-frequency vibration, adapting quickly to all external stimuli.

Palmar – the anterior surface or the palm of the hand.

Palpatory assessment – assessment through touching.

Papule – a small round, firm, elevated area in the skin, varying in size from a pinpoint to that of a small pea.

Parasympathetic nervous system or craniosacral outflow – an anabolic system that conserves the body's energy properties.

Parietal – pertaining to the walls of a cavity or an organ.

Parkinson's disease – a neurological disorder that is progressive and degenerative in nature. It is marked by the destruction of certain areas of the brain (specifically, dopamine-producing neurons) and depletion of the neurotransmitter dopamine.

Passive stretching – form of stretching where the client remains relaxed (passive) and the therapist applies the stretch.

Pathogen or pathogenic agent – a biological agent capable of causing disease.

Pectoral – pertaining to the thorax or chest area.

Pedal – referring to the foot.

Percussion or tapotement – a massage stroke which consists of repetitive, staccato, striking movements of the hands either simultaneously or alternately, with loose wrists and fingers, in order to stimulate the underlying tissue.

Pericarditis – an inflammation of the parietal pericardium that may be due to trauma or infection.

Periosteum – a fibrous dense vascular connective tissue sheath that surrounds the bone and penetrates the bone anchoring itself to the bone.

Peripheral – also referred to as superficial, the outside surface (periphery) or surround external area of a structure.

Peripheral nervous system – a portion of the nervous system that is composed of nerves emerging from the central nervous system.

Peritoneum – the largest serous membrane in the body that encompasses the entire abdominal wall. Sections of the peritoneum include the mesenteries, the parietal and visceral peritoneum, and the greater and lesser omentum.

Peritonitis – bacteria or irritating substances that enter the abdominal cavity causing an acute inflammation of the peritoneum.

Petrissage – a massage stroke that is a rhythmic lifting of the muscle tissue away from the bone or underlying structures, followed by firm kneading or squeezing the muscle followed by a release of tissue.

Phlebitis – is an inflammation of a vein accompanied by pain.

Plantar – the bottom surface of the foot.

Plexus – a network of nerves.

Polarity – is a form of bodywork that uses simple touch and gentle rocking.

Popliteal – posterior aspect of the knee.

Posterior or dorsal – referring to the back of a structure.

Prone – face down lying position.

Proprioceptive neuromuscular facilitation (PNF) – a therapy for rehabilitation of soft tissue disorders based on reciprocal inhibition relaxation. Also known as *contract-relax technique*.

Protocol – the form that describes the steps used in the therapy plan.

Proximal – nearer to the point of reference, usually toward the trunk of the body.

Psoriasis – red, flaky skin elevations marked by remissions and exacerbations.

Pulmonary edema – a disproportionate amount of blood and interstitial fluid in the lungs.

Range of motion (ROM) – a measurement of joint movement, which can be either active or passive.

Reciprocal inhibition (RI) – occurs when muscle acting on a joint contracts and the opposite muscle is reflexively inhibited.

Referred pain – pain illicited at a site distant from the injured or diseased body part.

Reflex arc – the functional component of the nervous system in which the sensory and motor neuron innervate a muscle, gland, or organ.

Renal – pertaining to the kidneys.

Sauna bath – a hot-air bath with temperatures ranging from 160 to 180° F in 6 to 8% humidity.

Schwann's cells – located in the peripheral nervous system that produce the myelin sheaths to axons.

Sciatica – a condition whereby the sciatic nerve is inflamed with resulting dull pain and tenderness in the buttock region with sharper pain or numbness radiating down the leg.

Scleroderma – an autoimmune disorder affecting blood vessels and connective tissue.

Scoliosis – is an abnormal lateral curvature of the spine.

Scope of practice – defines the working parameters of a particular profession. This may vary from state to state.

Seated position – a massage given to a client while they are seated. Also known as chair position. The client may be seated in an ordinary chair or one that is specially designed for client comfort.

Sebaceous or oil glands – glands that attach to hair follicles and possess ducts (exocrine). Sebum is secreted from sebaceous glands.

Senile lentigo – a condition found on older people whereby the skin has tan or brown patches. Found especially on those that have had excessive exposure to the sun.

Serous membranes – these membranes line closed body cavities and secrete a thin, fluid between the parietal and visceral layers, which lubricates organs and reduces friction between the organs in the thoracic or abdominopelvic cavities.

Shiatsu – is a general term for Japanese bodywork based on traditional meridian theory, in which *tsubo* (acupoints are pressed to balance the flow of energy or *Ki*.

Shingles – a reactivation of the latent herpes zoster (chickenpox) virus causing an acute infection of the peripheral nervous system.

Sitz bath – a sitting bath with warm water covering the hips and coming up to the navel. The design is such that the legs may remain out of the water.

Skeletal or voluntary muscle – nerve impulses must be present in order that these muscles may contract. They are muscles that attach to bones and their membranes, fascia and other muscles.

Skin pallor – refers to unnatural paleness or lack of skin color.

Sliding filament theory – the theory of how muscle filaments slide past each other in order to change muscle length.

Smooth visceral or involuntary muscle – muscles that line the walls of hollow organs. They are adapted to sustain long sustained contractions and use very little energy.

SOAP – an acronym for reporting. **S**ubjective assessment information, **O**bjective assessment information, **A**pplication of massage or therapy, and **P**lan course of action.

Somatic reflexes – reflexes responsible for the contraction of skeletal muscle (e.g., knee jerk or patella reflex).

Spasticity – increase muscle tone and stiffness associated with an increase in tendon reflexes.

Spina bifida – a congenital defect in which there is a malformation in the spine.

Spinal cord – the structure within the canal of the vertebral canal and is an extension of the brain stem from the foramen magnum to the region of L2.

Spinal nerves – the nerves that originate from the spinal cord.

Sprain – the stretching or tearing of the ligamentous structure of a joint, with associated pain, swelling, and possible disability.

Squamous cell carcinoma – a type of skin cancer. It begins as a scaly pigmented area that could develop into an ulcerated crater.

Static stretching – slow held stretches with no bouncing.

Steam bath or wet sauna – hot vapor baths in a specially designed chamber where temperatures are maintained at 105 to 130° F at 100% humidity.

Sterilization – a technique that uses heat, water, chemicals, or gases to destroy microorganisms.

Strain – a muscle or tendon injury caused by a violent contraction, forced stretching, or synergistic failure.

Stretching – lengthening or extending the muscle tissue to its full length.

Summation – occurs when a subthreshold stimulus is repeated in succession and cumulatively creates a nerve impulse.

Superior, cranial, or cephalic – situated above or toward the head.

Supine – lying face up.

Sympathetic nervous system or thoracolumbar outflow – a catabolic system that is involved with spending body resources and with preparing the body for emergency situations.

Synaptic transmission – the one-way bridging of the synaptic gap to convey the nerve impulse (from axon to dendrite) to the next neuron.

Synarthrotic joint – type of joint in which movement is absent or extremely limited.

Synovial fluid – viscous fluid that provides nutrition and lubrication to joints.

Synovial membrane – membranes that line joint cavities of freely moving joints. These membranes secrete synovial fluids.

Tachycardia – rapid heart rate (more than 100 beats per minute).

Temporal mandibular joint (TMJ) – a joint where the jawbone articulates with the temporal bone of the skull often causing pain and tenderness.

Tendinitis – inflammation of the tendon, accompanied by pain and swelling.

Tendon – tough fibrous connective tissue that attaches muscle to bone, fascia, or other connective tissue structures.

Testosterone – an androgenic hormone that promotes secondary male sex characteristics, as well as libido (sex drive) and sperm production.

Thermoreceptors – receptors sensitive to temperature changes located immediately under the skin.

Thoracic duct – the lymphatic duct that drains lymph from the parts of the body not drained by the right lymphatic duct.

Thyroxin – a hormone secreted by the thyroid gland that stimulates the metabolic rate of the body.

Tonus – a state of continuous, partial muscle contraction.

Topical – pertaining to the surface.

Torticollis – condition in which the head leans to one side because of neck muscle contractions (wry neck).

Touch – laying the hands on the skin.

Trager, Milton – founder of a method using gentle shaking to eliminate tension.

Transverse or horizontal plane – the plane that creates the superior and inferior sections.

Travell, Janet – founder of trigger points that cause myofascial pain.

Treatment record – a journal of treatment or therapy sessions that contain the client's information and SOAP forms for each session.

Trigger points – hypersensitive areas in muscles, fascia, tendons, and ligaments that refer pain to distal regions of the body.

Ulcer – a lesion in a membrane most commonly in parts of the digestive tract which is exposed to acidic gastric juices.

Universal donor – a donor with type O blood whereby their blood will not react to any other blood types.

Universal precautions – a health-preserving system that includes the following: handwashing, gloves, protective eyewear, nose-face masks, protective clothing, methods for laundering, cleaning and disinfecting equipment, and proper methods for disposing of used medical and biological material.

Universal recipient – recipient with type AB blood who can receive all other blood types.

Urinary incontinence – the inability to control micturition.

Varicose veins – dilated veins possessing incompetent valves.

Vasodilation – the diameter of a blood vessel becomes wider.

Veins – blood vessels that drain the tissues and organs and return blood back to the heart and lungs.

Vibration – a massage stroke that is a rapid shaking, trembling, or oscillating movement that is applied with full hands, fingertips, to induce relaxation.

Vodder, Emil – the founder of manual lymph drainage, which assists the flow of lymph through the vessels.

Yang – demonstrates the back of the body, the light, high, hot, outside, active, and excessive of the natural process and compliments Yin.

Yin – demonstrates the front of the body, the dark, low, cold, inside, passive, and deficiency of the natural process and compliments Yang, the opposite.